Healthy
COMPETITION

Healthy

COMPETITION

What's Holding Back Health Care and How to Free It

MICHAEL F. CANNON
& MICHAEL D. TANNER

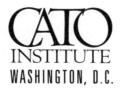

CATO
INSTITUTE
WASHINGTON, D.C.

Library of Congress Cataloging-in-Publication Data

Cannon, Michael F.

  Healthy competition : what's holding back health care and how to
free it, 2nd ed./ Michael F. Cannon & Michael D. Tanner.
    p. cm.
  Includes bibliographical references and index.
  ISBN 1-930865-81-3 (cloth : alk. paper)
    1. Medical care—United States. 2. Medical policy—United States.
  3. Health care reform—United States.   I. Tanner, Michael, 1956–
  II. Title.

RA395.A3C36 2007
362.1'0973—dc22

                                             2005050787

Cover design by Jon Meyers.

Printed in the United States of America.

CATO INSTITUTE
1000 Massachusetts Ave., N.W.
Washington, D.C. 20001
www.cato.org

Contents

Acknowledgments

We owe a debt of thanks to many people who helped this book along. Thanks go first to our dynamite research assistants, Adrienne Aldredge and Chris Gioffre, who tracked down much of the data herein. Thanks also to those whose comments on previous drafts strengthened the book considerably, including Peter Van Doren, Brink Lindsey, Bill Niskanen, Bob Helms, and Katie Jones, as well as to Debi Chakrabarty for her fact-checking skills. Thanks and empathy go to our editors, including Gene Healy and Micki Nussbaum. Whatever errors remain are ours alone. We would also like to thank Cato Institute president Ed Crane, executive vice president David Boaz, and George Shultz for their faith in this project.

Finally, we would like to thank our wives, Liz and Ellen, for alternating between being our toughest critics and our biggest fans.

Preface to the Second Edition

A great deal has happened since the Cato Institute published the first edition of *Healthy Competition* in 2005. The most obvious change was the Democratic takeover of Congress following the 2006 midterm elections. No sooner had the election results been calculated than Sen. Hillary Clinton (D-N.Y.) announced that Democrats would once again make health care reform a top legislative priority. "Health care is coming back," Senator Clinton said, adding, "It may be a bad dream for some."[1]

No one knows for certain what the new Democratic majority has in mind. But initial proposals regarding Medicaid and the Medicare prescription drug program are certainly steps in the direction of more government control over the medical marketplace. Rep. Pete Stark (D-Calif.), the new chairman of the Ways and Means Committee's Subcommittee on Health, introduced a bill calling for the creation of a Canadian-style single-payer system, as did Rep. John Dingell (D-Mich.), the new chairman of the Energy and Commerce Committee. In the Senate, Sen. Edward Kennedy (D-Mass.), perhaps the Senate's leading advocate of government-run health care, is the new chairman of the Health, Education, Labor and Pensions Committee. Many freshman Democrats also have called for some form of nationalized health insurance.

At the same time, many Republicans have abandoned their support for free markets. In Massachusetts, then-governor Mitt Romney (R) signed a law requiring all state residents to purchase health insurance and creating a regulatory scheme resembling the failed 1993 Clinton health care plan.[2] Meanwhile, in California, Gov. Arnold Schwarzenegger (R) put forward an even broader plan for universal coverage that would require individuals to purchase coverage, require employers to offer coverage, dramatically expand the state's Medicaid program, and increase taxes on health care providers.[3] Despite the tax increases on Californians, taxpayers in other states would pay more than three-fourths of the cost of Governor Schwarzenegger's plan.[4]

Yet, there have also been positive developments. Consumer-oriented health care plans continue to make inroads. For example, more than six million Americans now have health savings accounts (HSAs). And Congress recently liberalized some of the regulations surrounding HSAs, allowing account holders to make greater tax-free contributions.

Perhaps even more important, President George W. Bush has proposed a "standard health insurance deduction" that would eliminate the tax disparity between employer-provided and individually purchased health insurance. We discuss this proposal in Chapter 5 and conclude that it would be a dramatic improvement over HSAs. Variations of this proposal have long been recommended by serious health economists from across the political spectrum. Indeed, the president's proposal mirrors many aspects of the "large HSAs" concept we introduced in this book's first edition. For a sitting president to advance such a dramatic proposal marks a significant breakthrough in the debate over health care reform.

Why is health care reform receiving so much attention? Not only do the problems we described in 2005 persist, but many have deepened. Private health insurance grows more expensive. The cost of government health programs continues to climb and to threaten future generations with a crushing tax burden. The quality of medical care continues to suffer. Consumers still have precious little control over their health care dollars and decisions.

Indeed, health care reform is poised to be a dominant issue in the 2008 presidential campaign. Early contenders for the Democratic presidential nomination have unanimously agreed that the next president should push for universal health insurance. Candidates such as former senator John Edwards (D-N.C.) and Gov. Bill Richardson (D-N.M.) advanced specific reform proposals as early as March 2007.[5]

It is our hope that this updated edition of *Healthy Competition* can inform that debate and give reformers the tools they will need to make health care of ever-increasing quality available to an ever-increasing number of Americans.

Michael F. Cannon
Michael D. Tanner

Foreword

George P. Shultz

We begin with a riddle. What country's health care system offers the best health services in the world, is constantly criticized for not being accessible enough, and yet is so accessible that overutilization is leading to runaway costs? The first part reveals the answer could only be America. The remainder gives the contours of a paradox that vexes policymakers year in and year out. Welcome to health care, American-style. Untangling these apparent inconsistencies is an essential step in gearing our health system to the emerging modern world.

What are some of the characteristics of this modern world? For one thing, increased longevity, aging baby boomers, and new medical technologies presage greater use of medical care. Take demography. Our population's age structure is changing. The baby boomers are about to start moving into the over-65 category, while longevity keeps increasing. We are getting older as well as healthier, or maybe, because we are healthier, we are getting older. Nevertheless, the older we are, the closer we are to death, and a disproportionate share of health care spending comes toward the end of a person's life. Moreover, innovation enables modern medicine to satisfy needs that yesterday went unmet, which draws more resources into the health sector.

These trends are colliding with a health care system that already encourages overutilization. To a greater degree than even our neighbors to the north, Americans rely on someone else to pay for their health care—a tradition that had its inception in the World War II era. Employers needed workers, and the only enticement they could offer that was not subject to wartime wage and price controls was health benefits. Providing health insurance was a no-brainer for employers, but no one should be surprised that when the marginal cost of health care approaches zero, utilization skyrockets.

Entitlement programs add fuel to the fire. For example, Medicare is essentially "free" fee-for-service health care for the elderly. Seniors, even the well-to-do, pay few if any copayments. Dr. John E. Wennberg of Dartmouth has been studying regional variations in Medicare health care claims since 1967 and, more recently, their effects on health outcomes. Wennberg shows that about one-third of all health care purchased by Medicare is unnecessary—and some is possibly harmful. Life expectancy is no greater in regions that receive more intensive medical care, and Medicare surveys find that their quality of care is no better. A summary of Wennberg's research concludes: "The difference in lifetime Medicare spending between a typical 65-year-old in Miami and one in Minneapolis is more than $50,000, equivalent to a new Lexus GS 400 with all the trimmings." Such large inefficiencies suggest we could maintain—or even improve upon—current levels of productivity at a much lower cost. How?

America's health care system needs to give consumers more responsibility and more control over their health care expenditures. Many authoritative studies show that consumer control can reduce costs drastically without any negative impact on health outcomes. The RAND Health Insurance Experiment demonstrated that as copayments increase, utilization goes down but health outcomes stay the same. (Read more about this experiment in Chapter 4 of this fascinating book.) The consumer-directed health care movement—with health savings accounts at the helm—is already hard at work ascertaining how to provide patients greater value for the dollar. The Cato Institute played a leading role in bringing health savings accounts to workers, and this new option is growing in popularity every day. In these pages, Michael Cannon and Michael Tanner build on that tradition and show that expanding health savings accounts can give consumers control over all of their health care dollars.

Consumer-directed health care has its detractors. Do consumers care enough to become informed? Do they have the capacity to understand health alternatives and to make intelligent choices?

Overwhelmingly, the evidence answers in the affirmative. Ordinary Americans are increasingly on the ball when it comes to their health. In fact, markets are already recognizing and meeting consumers' demand for accessible health care and more health information.

For example, in some retail stores, nurse stations with basic equipment can provide you with quick diagnoses of ordinary problems for a small fee. WebMD, an online resource of medical information, receives an average of 889,000 visitors daily. Forrester Research reports that baby boomers are better educated and more affluent than previous generations, and are considerably more comfortable with technology. These rising seniors are using the Internet en masse for health and leisure activities. European consumers too are increasingly likely to seek health information online.

Accustomed to serving themselves on retail and media sites, consumers hunger for useful online content and comparative evaluation tools from their health care providers. A growing wave of health care consumerism among young, health-conscious individuals is setting the stage for consumer-directed health plans (CDHP). Plans that are slow in developing a CDHP risk losing healthier, engaged consumers to rival plans. The more of a stake consumers have in their spending decisions, the better informed and the more demanding they will be.

Yet America needs more than just health savings accounts. To carry the health care debate on its next lap, America first needs a clear, well-informed, and well-reasoned analysis of the apparent paradox of its health care system. And it needs an agenda for reform that respects the wonders that modern medicine has developed and the creative market processes that deliver them. On the following pages, Cannon and Tanner offer proposals that would further tap the power of markets to make health care more valuable and more affordable. That makes *Healthy Competition* essential reading.

Introduction: What Can Competition Do for Patients?

Health care in the United States is not what it should be. For one thing, it seems to grow less affordable each year. Official reports tell us that prices for medical care consistently rise faster than prices for nonmedical items. In particular, health insurance premiums are rising faster than both inflation and earnings, and are thus taking up a growing share of family budgets. Without health insurance, families risk enormous medical bills in the event of serious illness or injury. Yet tens of millions of Americans have no health insurance, either because it has become too expensive or isn't worth the price. Government spending adds a number of very large (if somewhat hidden) items to the nation's health care bill.

The burden of paying for health care is only part of the problem. It also seems that health care quality is not always as high as it should be. America is a leader in medical innovation. Many Americans receive the best care available anywhere in the world, and many foreigners visit America to take advantage of cutting-edge medicine. However, a surprising number of patients receive substandard care. Substandard treatment can actually increase costs—both the costs associated with prolonged illness and the costs of additional care. Uneven quality—high quality in some areas, lower quality in others—seems to persist over time, in part due to a lack of information on providers and services. Employers, insurers, and government officials are just now beginning to take notice of the fact that substandard care may be partly responsible for rising health care costs.

Furthermore, patients seem to be losing control over their health care decisions. Health care is not like other goods and services. It exists to extend life and reduce pain. Many patients would value being able to make their own health care decisions, with the advice of their doctors, more than they value being able to choose their own cars, car insurance, or computers. Yet Americans have fewer choices when it comes to health insurance than they do with car

1

insurance. Employers have been making decisions about Americans' health insurance for as long as anyone can remember. Government also makes many health insurance decisions for consumers, particularly senior citizens. In recent years, employers and insurance companies have begun making what amount to treatment decisions as well. Managed care probably does eliminate some unnecessary costs. But patients resent the lack of choice this entails, and doctors resent the intrusion on their professional judgment. Impediments to patient choice crop up in other corners of the medical marketplace, such as laws that prevent terminally ill patients from choosing their own courses of treatment.

These are vexing problems. Quality, affordability, and choice seem to present tradeoffs: getting more of one seems to involve getting less of the others. On the one hand, employers, insurance companies, and government can set limits on what treatments they will cover. This may eliminate low-quality care. But it also reduces patient choice and would sometimes block access to necessary care. On the other hand, if patients are given free rein, what's to prevent them from overutilizing the health care system or choosing low-quality care and imposing costs on everyone else?

How can high-quality health care be made affordable, without sacrificing patient choice? That is a question asked over and over again in health policy circles. It underlies debates over health insurance, prescription drugs, primary and preventive care, hospital care, and aid to the poor. And it has stumped policymakers in Washington and the state capitols for generations. The thesis of this book is that the way to find solutions to the vexing problems of America's health care system is through a competitive market process. We do not claim to know any particular solution to these problems. We do, however, propose a method of discovering them.

Why Competition?

Competition is a tool for finding answers we don't have. At the beginning of each baseball season, opinions run strong about which club has assembled the strongest team. But we do not know, and will not know, which team is the best until the regular season, playoffs, and World Series winnow the field to one. (Even then, there can be passionate disagreement over the result. That is why we have *next* season.) Competition puts to the test both the product (the ball club) and people's opinions ("The Cubs will win the pennant this year—I guarantee it").

If we had answers instead of just opinions, competition would be unnecessary. As the late Nobel laureate Friedrich Hayek wrote, "In sporting events . . . it would be patently absurd to sponsor a contest if we knew in advance who the winner would be."[1] The reverse is also true: it would be silly to hang a gold medal on someone because we believe she is the fastest runner. Without a race, how could we know? It is the race that gives us the answer; the contest tells us what we want to know.

The same is true of scientific discovery. It would make little sense to ordain that Newtonian physics is the only way to understand the universe and to forbid competing theories. Nor would it make sense to allow only one person or school to offer and test such theories. What if the ordained theory or scientists were wrong? And how would we know whether they were wrong without allowing others to offer criticism and alternative theories? In science, the truth emerges in time through a competitive process. "Competition," Hayek explained, "must be seen as a process in which people acquire and communicate knowledge."[2] Competition is how society acknowledges that it does not have the information it wants, and demonstrates that it is serious about discovering it.

Competition plays a special role in economics, including health care. Scientific discovery typically pursues immutable, unchanging facts. Economic competition searches for information and answers that are constantly changing. What is the best way to lower the price of health care and increase quality? How many doctors does the United States need? Or hospitals? Or magnetic resonance imaging (MRI) machines? In what parts of the country are these most needed? What should the prices be for MRI services? Can some tasks that are usually performed by physicians be performed as reliably by other medical professionals? What is the best way to ensure that drugs are safe and effective? Where should drug manufacturers focus their research? The answers to these questions change constantly as technological advances, demographics, and other factors produce changes in available resources and societal needs.

As a result, Hayek argued, finding the answers to economic questions is an ongoing process requiring constant experimentation and learning. Unlike a footrace, economic competition never quite arrives at a final answer. It keeps revealing the new "best" answer in an ever-changing world. Economic competition is not merely the bustle of greedy businessmen trying to make a buck, although it certainly can be that. More important, Hayek wrote, it is "a discovery procedure" that constantly provides and adjusts information that we cannot know, and therefore cannot use, without a competitive process.[3]

What has to be in place for market competition to provide us with these answers? First and foremost, market competition requires a wide pool of competitors and potential competitors, including entrepreneurs with new ideas. Finding the answers to the prior vexing questions requires capturing and using knowledge as diverse and dispersed as

- whether patients are waiting too long to see specialists in Tallahassee,
- what type of health coverage matters most to the near-elderly in Spokane, and
- how to make primary care hassle-free.

These bits of information—and ideas on how to use them—are scattered across vast numbers of people. Therefore, individuals must have maximum latitude to apply their knowledge and ideas to meet these changing needs. Open competition gives entrepreneurs that latitude, and thus calls forth information and ideas from all corners. That suggests that competitive health care markets should have low barriers to entry, and that entrepreneurs should have the flexibility to experiment with new ideas.

Second, a competitive market needs some mechanism to evaluate each producer's ideas and efforts. Such a mechanism is most useful if it constantly feeds information to each producer about how much value she is providing consumers. The obvious feedback mechanism is consumers themselves.

Information about available health care resources is dispersed among millions of producers and potential producers. Likewise, information about what consumers value is stored in the minds of hundreds of millions of consumers. Allowing consumers to make their own health care decisions is a way of capturing and conveying that information. When consumers are free to choose the health care services they want, that information is transmitted to both favored and disfavored producers through the customer's purchasing decision. Individual choice is particularly important when we consider that different people have different values. When economic decisions are made by a mechanism other than individual choice, many consumers' preferences will go unnoticed and their needs unmet.

Having consumers weigh different options against one another is a necessary part of discovering what consumers value. If consumers can choose only one of two options, they will choose the one that provides them the most value. That information is then captured and used by producers. But if patients have their freedom of choice taken away, or are allowed to consume medical care for "free," things change. In such cases, the market cannot learn what they value most. If they face no tradeoffs, they likely will consume medical care that they do not value very much. Those resources are then not available to meet other social needs. A competitive health care market needs consumers who are free to choose from competing options and who face tradeoffs among competing options.

When these conditions of a competitive market are met, individual choice actually promotes lower prices and higher quality. Since consumers desire both, they will naturally choose the combination of health insurance and medical services that gives them the best mix of both. When innovations come along that provide greater value— that is, higher quality and/or lower prices—consumers will gravitate toward those new options. The result is a market process that makes health care of ever-increasing quality available to an ever-increasing number of consumers.

Unfortunately, when it comes to health care, government has long behaved as if it knows all the answers. Through laws and regulations, it has claimed that it knows the best way to provide medical care for workers in their retirement. It has picked one form of private health insurance that should be favored before all others. It claims that it knows the only way to protect the public from unsafe medical technologies, and that it knows the best way to finance medical care for the needy.

Year after year, government continues to choose "winners" in the medical marketplace. Each time it does, it hampers the competitive process that reduces costs and increases quality. People often claim that government must step in because a particular question is too important to be put to the test of competition. (Often, the same people have a personal interest in what they claim is the "right" answer.) Nonetheless, even when entry, innovation, consumer choice, and market valuation are hampered, competition relentlessly tries to break through its restraints.

Competition and Health Care

The evidence is all around us. In markets where consumers are free to choose from numerous producers, competition reduces prices and makes products of ever-increasing quality available to an ever-increasing number of consumers. Michael E. Porter of Harvard University and Elizabeth Teisberg of the University of Virginia write,

> In healthy competition, relentless improvements in processes and methods drive down costs. Product and service quality rise steadily. Innovation leads to new and better approaches, which diffuse widely and rapidly. Uncompetitive providers are restructured or go out of business. Value-adjusted prices fall, and the market expands. This is the trajectory common to all well-functioning industries—computers, mobile communications, banking, and many others.[4]

However, they continue,

> Health could not be more different. Costs are high and rising, despite efforts to reduce them, and these rising costs cannot be explained by improvements in quality. Quite the opposite: Medical services are restricted or rationed, many patients receive care that lags currently accepted procedures or standards, and high rates of preventable medical error persist.[5]

Porter's and Teisberg's description of health care markets is accurate, although not uniformly. In health care markets where consumer choice and competition are free to operate, they deliver higher quality and lower prices just as they do in other markets.

Consider drugs, for example. A study by University of Pennsylvania economist Patricia Danzon found that prices for generic drugs are typically lower in the United States than in eight other advanced nations, while over-the-counter drugs are "considerably cheaper" in the United States. Danzon attributes that to "the relatively unregulated, more competitive structure of the U.S. market."[6] Although Danzon finds that pioneer drugs are more expensive in the United States (at least while under patent), a study by Tufts University finds

Figure 1
AVERAGE PRICE FOR LASIK SURGERY, 1999–2004 (ONE EYE)

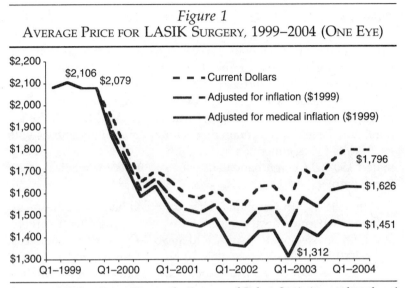

SOURCES: Market Scope Research, Bureau of Labor Statistics, and authors' calculations.

that when multiple drugs are approved for the same indication, competition dramatically lowers the cost of those drugs as well. Cholesterol-lowering statins introduced in 2003 cost 45 percent less than those introduced 10 years earlier. Anti-hypertensive drugs introduced in the mid-1990s cost 72 percent less than those introduced in the early 1980s.[7]

Cosmetic surgery is another area where choice and competition deliver higher quality and lower prices. In that market, patients pay directly and therefore must weigh the costs and benefits of each procedure. As a result, inflation-adjusted prices have fallen every year from 1992 to 2001.[8]

Patients also weigh the costs and benefits of laser eye surgery, another highly competitive market where prices have fallen dramatically. As Figure 1 demonstrates, the average price for Lasik surgery in 1999 was about $2,100 per eye. Within two years, it had fallen to less than $1,600 per eye.[9] Many patients pay less.[10] The price of refractive surgery dropped even more relative to overall inflation and medical inflation. Were Figure 1 to adjust for quality improvements—a driving factor behind recent price increases—it would

7

show that average prices have fallen even more dramatically. It is also notable that these falling prices occur despite the fact that more than 80 percent of Lasik patients search for an experienced surgeon with a strong reputation, rather than just the lowest price.[11]

Consumer choice and competition are even making urgent medical care more accessible. In a growing trend,[12] hospitals in such countries as Argentina, Barbados, Costa Rica, India, Malaysia, Singapore, and Thailand are competing with hospitals in countries with long waits for treatment or high health care costs. In 2003, an estimated 150,000 foreign patients traveled to India for medical care.[13] For example,

- In 2004, North Carolinian Howard Staab had no health insurance when his doctor told him he needed open-heart surgery. Durham Regional Hospital told Staab the procedure would cost $200,000. Instead, Staab flew to New Delhi where Dr. Naresh Trehan—formerly a professor at New York University Medical School—performed the operation at Escorts Heart Institute and Research Center for less than $10,000.[14]
- Tom Raudaschl, a mountain guide and Canadian resident suffering from osteoarthritis, found he would have to wait as many as three years for a hip resurfacing operation in Canada or pay $21,000 for the procedure in the United States. Apollo Hospitals in Chennai, India, performed the operation for less than $5,000.[15] The same choice spared Terry Salo of British Columbia a painful year's wait for hip replacement surgery.[16]
- Robert Beeney, "a 64-year-old real estate consultant from San Francisco," paid $6,600 for a hip joint resurfacing in Hyderabad, India. The procedure was not covered by his health insurance and would have cost him $25,000 at home.[17]
- To obtain coronary bypass surgery from the National Health Service in his native England, 73-year-old George Marshall would have had to wait more than six months. At a private British hospital, the procedure would have cost him $38,000. Marshall commented, "At 73, I don't have the time to wait . . . Six months could be the rest of my life." Instead, Marshall underwent surgery in Bangalore, India. The total cost including travel expenses was $8,400. Marshall remarked that under Britain's NHS, "you are just a number," while at Bangalore's Wockhardt Hospital, "you are a person."[18]

Foreign hospitals aggressively compete with each other (and U.S. hospitals) on the basis of price and quality. Apollo promises what one report describes as "First World health care at Third World prices."[19] Cardiac and orthopedic surgeries often cost one-fifth to one-quarter the U.S. price, more than enough to cover the cost of airfare and lodging (which some hospitals will arrange).[20] In Indian hospitals, orthopedic procedures cost one-fourth, and cataract surgery can cost one-tenth, the price in U.S. hospitals.[21] Dr. Trehan claims that Escorts charges $60 for an MRI, compared with $700 in New York.[22]

Trehan also claims his Escorts Heart Institute and Research Center posts lower death rates from heart surgery than New York-Presbyterian Hospital, where former president Bill Clinton received bypass surgery. The reason? "Our surgeons are much better."[23] A British-trained pediatrician in India's Apollo Hospitals commented, "Nobody even questions the capability of an Indian doctor, because there isn't a big hospital in the United States where there isn't an Indian doctor working."[24]

International competition is also lowering the cost of processing health insurance claims, interpreting the results of diagnostic tests, and conducting clinical trials for new drugs.[25]

Here at home, competition delivers similar results—where it can be found. A study by Stanford University economists Mark McClellan (now the head of Medicare and Medicaid) and Daniel Kessler found that in the 1990s "competition among hospitals was unambiguously welfare-improving." Compared with less competitive markets, the cost of treating heart attack patients in competitive hospital markets was lower, readmission rates were lower, and survival rates were higher. The authors found that "competition had the potential to improve [heart attack] mortality by 4.4 percent" and suggested that competition likely produced similar benefits in other areas of hospital care.[26]

In a subsequent study, Kessler and Jeffrey Geppert found that greater competition between hospitals leads to a better match of resources to needs. Severely ill heart attack patients receive more intensive care in competitive hospital markets than they do in less competitive markets, and those treated in less competitive markets "have significantly worse health outcomes." When it comes to less severely ill heart attack victims, however, something changes. Those patients receive more intensive treatment in less competitive markets than they do in more competitive markets. Yet the added expense produces no improvement in health outcomes.[27] Kessler and Geppert's findings suggest that competition eliminates unnecessary costs and moves resources to avenues where they are needed and where they will deliver results.

In these examples, competition is lowering prices and improving quality. Why are these successes the exception and not the rule? The answer is that in America's health care sector, a dense thicket of laws and regulations disables the competitive process that produces such outcomes. Government discourages patients from shopping for value and encourages them to disregard costs. It pays doctors and hospitals according to volume with no regard to quality. It restricts the choices available to patients and blocks competition among providers of medical goods and services. Through tax policy, subsidies, and regulation, government reduces patients' freedom to choose, reduces competition, and obstructs the market processes that deliver higher quality at lower prices.

Even where competition *can* be found in America's health care system, Porter and Teisberg argue, much of it takes place at the wrong level. Instead of providers competing for patients, one finds health plans, hospitals, and provider networks competing for the business of bureaucracies that purchase care on behalf of patients. A major report by the Federal Trade Commission and Department of Justice confirms that competition in the U.S. health care system is badly hampered:

> Competition has affected health care markets substantially over the past three decades. New forms of organization have developed in response to pressures for lower costs, and new strategies for lowering costs and enhancing quality have emerged. Nonetheless, competition remains less effective than possible in most health care markets, because the prerequisites for fully competitive markets are not fully satisfied.[28]

The agencies recommend encouraging patients to become more prudent health care consumers; realigning the self-interest of providers with patients' interest in low-cost, high-quality care; reducing government barriers to competition among medical professionals and facilities (e.g., hospitals); removing barriers to interstate competition;

targeting government subsidies directly to patients; and reducing regulations that increase the cost of health insurance.

Many take America's high and rising health care costs as a sign that health care is a special case in which consumer choice and competition do not work. Stanford University's Alain Enthoven has written, "A free market does not and cannot work in health insurance and health care . . . If not corrected by a careful design, this market is plagued by problems of . . . market failure."[29] Yale University professor George Silver, who was deputy assistant secretary for health under former president Lyndon B. Johnson, writes, "Today's dysfunctional health care system is a palpable example of the lessons that come from our national obsession with markets at all costs."[30]

Yet this view fails to account for the pervasive influence of government in the U.S. health care sector, and how that influence stifles market competition. According to Danzon, "Government is more pervasive in health care than in almost any other industry."[31] By at least one measure—the share of expenditures financed directly by patients—health care in the United States is more socialized than in other nations with explicitly socialized health care systems. Government directly finances health care for more than one-quarter of the U.S. population (77 million people in 2003),[32] or nearly half of all health expenditures. It heavily influences all other medical expenditures, sets prices and other terms for countless health care transactions, and prevents many exchanges and arrangements that would benefit both parties, either through outright prohibitions or by refusing to uphold contracts. Columbia University law professor William Sage notes that many have "ignored this reality and indulged the belief that U.S. health care is a private system governed by private competition."[33]

The fact that the United States still has the most market-oriented health care system among advanced countries says more about how little other nations rely on choice and competition in health care than about how much the United States does so.

Competition vs. Controls

America faces a choice between two approaches to meeting the nation's medical needs: greater choice and competition in an open marketplace, or more government control. Ultimately, the decision

11

is between competing visions of whether power in the medical marketplace should reside with individuals or with government.

In December 2003, President George W. Bush signed into law a piece of legislation that embodied both options. Beginning in 2006, the "Medicare Modernization Act" will add outpatient prescription drug subsidies to the Medicare program, taxing working Americans to provide prescription drugs to the elderly and disabled. This legislation represents the largest expansion of government influence in the health care arena in 40 years. With the stroke of a pen, President Bush imposed unfunded obligations on current and future taxpayers that are greater than the unfunded obligations of the entire Social Security program (see Chapter 6).

While the new Medicare prescription drug subsidies will reduce choice and competition in one area of America's health care sector, health savings accounts (HSAs) will restore these natural market forces in another. The Medicare Modernization Act created HSAs beginning in January 2004. HSAs represent a milestone in health care policy, for they help restore the right to choose one's doctor and one's health insurance, to own one's health insurance policy, and to save for future medical needs. HSAs replace the perverse incentives involved in paying providers on the basis of volume with sensible incentives that result from paying providers on the basis of value. HSAs encourage providers to compete for individual patients rather than health plans and networks, as Porter and Teisberg recommend. HSAs represent a significant departure from the prevailing culture of health care in America, focusing producers' attention on the needs of consumers, and all parties on the need for greater economy and innovation.

Although a modest reform on their own, HSAs have revolutionary implications. They return government health policy to what must be its first principle: the right of individuals to make their own health decisions. Yet fully restoring the freedom of patients and doctors requires more than health savings accounts. Fulfilling this vision requires respecting the right of Americans to choose for themselves:

- whether to purchase health insurance and what type;
- how to finance their health care needs in retirement, rather than be forced into a government-controlled scheme;

- how to assist the medically needy, rather than be forced to finance often unnecessary and harmful "charity" care;
- whether to try an experimental treatment;
- what type of medical professional to consult; and
- whether to choose a different level of malpractice protection than courts would apply.

It also requires respecting the right of medical professionals to choose their areas of practice, to run their practices as they choose, and to innovate, all free from unnecessary government obstacles.

The principles of consumer choice and competition that underlie health savings accounts can be applied to all areas of the medical marketplace: the taxation of health expenditures, government subsidies, regulation of medical providers and products, and the medical liability system. In each of these areas, lawmakers should increase the number of decisions made by individuals and decrease the number of decisions made by government officials. This includes removing outright restrictions on the freedom of patients, providers, and taxpayers, as well as laws that reward or punish Americans for the decisions they make about their health care. The key principles can be distilled down into two maxims:

(1) Congress shall make no law encouraging or hindering particular methods of medical care, or of financing medical care.
(2) The right of the people to contract for medical goods and services shall not be infringed.

Past patients' rights legislation has consumed reams of paper in an effort to restrict the number of choices individuals may make about their health care. These maxims have a different goal: to expand the choices available to patients, and to affirm the patient's right to choose. Health savings accounts represent a first step toward this vision of a free-market health care system.

The alternative vision would restrict freedom by maintaining or expanding government influence over America's health care sector in the pursuit of greater health, equity, or consumer protection. Though usually well-intentioned, measures that expand government's influence often achieve the opposite of these goals. Worse, this vision produces harms that reach beyond the realm of economics or even that of health. It demeans the dignity and diversity of the

American people for government to deny them the freedom to care for their minds and bodies according to their own judgment.

A health care system free of any special involvement by government will give pause to many. To some extent, health care is a special area of public policy. In many instances, it is essential for survival. Americans oppose the idea that some people might suffer because they cannot afford medical care. Many Americans believe government must play a special role to protect patients from the errors and predations of health care practitioners and corporations.

Yet government's presence in the medical marketplace extends far beyond what can be justified by the desire to help in hard cases. By hindering the competitive process, government actually makes it more difficult for the medically needy to obtain care. Americans' aversion to allowing the needy to go without medical care is an indication both of the American people's compassion *and* what America might achieve with a health care system free of unnecessary government influence. Ultimately, the very fact that health care is often a matter of life or death is the most powerful argument for reducing government's influence over its provision. This is one of the themes that the remainder of this book explores.

This book is organized as follows. Part I examines the state of America's health care system, acknowledging the things it does well, dispelling certain popular misconceptions, and finally addressing some of the real problems it faces. Part II criticizes "reforms" that undoubtedly would make these existing problems worse. Part III examines how government influence has made America's health care sector what it is, and proposes ways of reducing government influence. We conclude with an outlook for the future, and the role that health savings accounts can play.

PART I

THE STATE OF AMERICA'S HEALTH CARE SYSTEM

1. What's Right

As noted earlier, many critics of free markets conclude America's health care system demonstrates that free markets are an inferior way of providing medical care. Though inaccurate, this misperception is based on a partial truth. More than any other developed nation, America relies on private institutions and market mechanisms to deliver medical care. The harmful effects of government influence are significant, yet the successes of America's relatively market-oriented approach to health care bear mentioning.

Innovation

By many measures, the United States has the finest health care system in the world. Most of the world's top doctors, hospitals, and research facilities are located in the United States. In the past 10 years, 14 of 25 recipients of the Nobel Prize for Medicine have been U.S. citizens. Four more practice in the United States.[1] American research and development, particularly in the pharmaceutical field, has produced the majority of medical breakthroughs over the past 50 years. Of the 152 major medicines introduced worldwide over the past 20 years, U.S. companies developed nearly half.[2] Eight of the 10 top-selling drugs worldwide in 2002 were produced by U.S. firms, and Americans played a key role in eight of the ten most important medical advances in the past 30 years.[3]

Nearly every type of advanced medical technology or procedure is more abundant in the United States than anywhere else in the world. Figure 1.1 shows the relative availability of technologies such as magnetic resonance imaging (MRI) units and computed tomography (CT) scanners on a per capita basis in various countries.[4]

If you are diagnosed with a significant illness, the United States is the place you want to be. For example, cancer patients are less likely to die from the disease in the United States than in other countries. Figure 1.2 shows the mortality-to-incidence ratios for breast, prostate, and colon cancers, as well as AIDS. The United States also seems to fare well in comparison to other nations when it comes to treating heart attacks and lung cancer.[5]

17

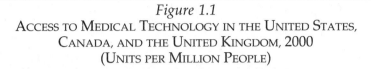

Figure 1.1
ACCESS TO MEDICAL TECHNOLOGY IN THE UNITED STATES,
CANADA, AND THE UNITED KINGDOM, 2000
(UNITS PER MILLION PEOPLE)

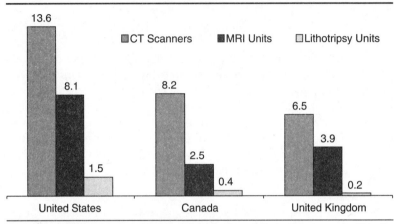

SOURCES: John Goodman et al., *Lives at Risk*; Gerard F. Anderson et al., "It's the Prices, Stupid: Why the United States Is So Different from Other Countries"; and Stephen Pollard, "European Health Care Consensus Group Paper."

It should come as no surprise, then, that patients all over the world seeking advanced medical care come to the United States for treatment. One U.S. hospital alone, the Mayo Clinic, treats roughly 7,200 foreigners every year. Johns Hopkins University Medical Center treats more than 6,000.[6] Nearly one-third of Canada's doctors have sent a patient abroad for treatment,[7] often to the United States, and Canadian governments and patients spend more than $1 billion every year on medical care in the United States.[8]

Common Misperceptions

Despite its strengths and consensus about some of its shortcomings, persistent misperceptions abound in debates over America's health care system. Perhaps the most prevalent is that America spends more on health care than other advanced nations but gets less in return. There is truth to this criticism as well: America does spend more on medical care than other countries, in both absolute and per·capita terms, and much of that spending is wasted. The reasons America likely spends too much on health care, why we

Figure 1.2
MORTALITY-TO-INCIDENCE RATIOS, VARIOUS ILLNESSES & NATIONS

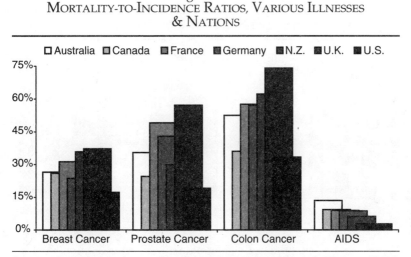

SOURCE: Gerard F. Anderson, Varduhi Petrosyan, and Peter S. Hussey, "Multinational Comparisons of Health Systems Data, 2002," Commonwealth Fund, October 2002, pp. 55–62; and Anderson and Hussey, "Multinational Comparisons of Health Systems Data," Commonwealth Fund, October 2000, pp. 17–18.

often get less than full value for our health care dollar, and some remedies are discussed later. It is important first to refine the critique by examining the first part of this myth: that spending more than other nations is in itself undesirable. In fact, high levels of medical spending are often a good thing. The second half of this myth— that other nation's health care systems outperform America's—is also worth debunking.

Is Spending More Necessarily Bad?

The United States has, by far, the most expensive health care system in the world, whether measured as a percentage of gross domestic product (GDP) or as expenditure per capita. As a percentage of GDP, U.S. health care spending (16 percent in 2005)[9] is more than six percentage points higher than the average of other industrialized countries (Figure 1.3).[10] Overall health care costs have outpaced GDP growth by more than four percentage points, on average, in the last five years and now total $2 trillion per year[11]—more than

19

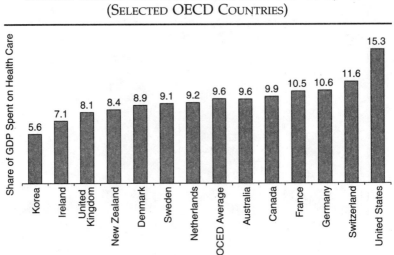

Figure 1.3
HEALTH CARE SPENDING AS A PERCENTAGE OF GDP, 2004
(SELECTED OECD COUNTRIES)

SOURCE: *OECD Health Data 2006*, October 10, 2006, "Total Expenditure on Health, % GDP."

consumers spent on housing, food, or automobiles, and more than the federal government spent on national defense.[12]

There are a number of reasons why high levels of health care spending should not be troubling or should even be seen as positive. Health care is considered a "normal good," meaning that spending is positively correlated with income. As income rises, people tend to demand more health care. The amount Americans spend on health care is to a large degree a reflection of America's wealth. Princeton University economist Uwe Reinhardt and scholars at Johns Hopkins University found that 90 percent of the variation in health spending among OECD nations "can be explained simply by GDP per capita." All by itself, America's high per capita GDP is enough to make its per capita health spending higher than any other OECD nation's, and accounts for 47 percent of the difference in per capita spending between the U.S. and the OECD median.[13]

An aging population also contributes to higher levels of health care spending. Gains in life expectancy increase that part of the population that consumes the most medical care (the elderly).

Figure 1.4
BENEFITS OF SPENDING AN ADDITIONAL $1 ON SELECTED
TREATMENTS

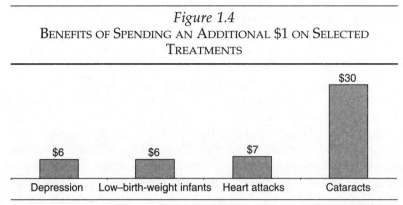

SOURCE: David M. Cutler and Mark McClellan, "Is Technological Change in Medicine Worth It?" *Health Affairs*, Vol. 20, No. 5, September/October 2001, pp. 11–29.

Technological advances in medical care also contribute to rising health care expenditures. Advances in medical care enable providers to aid patients for whom they could previously do little. Such advances call forth additional spending because they improve and lengthen lives. "The sickest person in the economy in 2002 is much more costly to treat than the sickest person in 1950 because technological progress has significantly shifted out the frontier medical condition that can be treated," writes U. C. Berkeley economist Charles Jones.[14]

Mark McClellan and Harvard University economist David M. Cutler posit that the benefits of technological advances overwhelm the added costs. They estimate that advances in technology meant that every additional dollar spent on treating heart attacks in the 1980s yielded the equivalent of $7 worth of increased longevity and quality of life. Advances in the treatment of depression and even expensive new treatments for low-birth-weight infants yield benefits worth six times the cost. And every dollar spent on cataract surgery yields more than $30 in benefits for patients who live an additional five years, and greater benefits among those who live longer (see Figure 1.4). Frank Lichtenberg of Columbia University estimates that from 1980 to 1992, every additional dollar spent on pharmaceuticals was associated with a $3.65 reduction in hospital expenditures.[15] Lichtenberg also estimates that the benefit-cost ratio of general medical expenditures is nearly 14 to 1 while the ratio for pharmaceutical research and development is more than 100 to 1.[16] Mark Duggan and William Evans of the University of Maryland found that anti-AIDS drugs introduced in the 1990s were cost-effective despite a threefold increase in Medicaid spending on HIV patients.[17] In these and many other cases, new technologies led to higher health care spending. Yet the additional spending often reduced the costs borne by patients.

Improvements in cardiac catheterization enable patients with heart disease to be treated younger, return to work faster, and live longer.[18] Increased availability of pacemakers and commercial defibrillators has also contributed to a significant reduction in deaths due to heart disease. Lichtenberg estimates new drugs account for as much as 40 percent of the increase in longevity in 52 nations from 1986 to 2000.[19] Jones estimates that between one-half and three-quarters of the growth in medical care expenditures from 1960 to 1997 was due to medical advances that enabled patients to get more per dollar spent.[20] "Technology often leads to more spending," Cutler and McClellan write, "but outcomes improve by even more."[21]

At the same time, technology often lowers prices. The inflation- and quality-adjusted price of treating heart attacks *declined* at a rate of just over 1 percent each year from 1983 to 1994.[22] Other studies have found similar effects with prices for cataract surgery[23] and depression.[24]

These productivity gains do not mean that America's medical marketplace is devoid of waste. Expensive new pharmaceuticals are often prescribed to patients who would do just as well with less expensive alternatives. Or waste may occur in routine, preventive, or other areas of medical care, such as unnecessary diagnostic tests or patients obtaining treatment in an emergency room rather than a less expensive clinic. In Chapters 4–6, we discuss how America's health care sector wastes billions of dollars and some of the reasons why. However, large productivity gains do suggest that much of America's health care spending is not wasted but is in fact very well spent. "Even if you take all the waste out of health care," Cutler notes, "the spending would still go up because we have a technology-intensive system that will continue and is delivering a lot of benefits in terms of longer, healthier lives."[25]

A final reason that high health expenditures need not be problematic has to do with America's leading role in medical innovation.

As the 2004 *Economic Report of the President* notes, "while all countries can benefit from research and development expenditures made by a single country, only the health expenditures in the innovating country will include the costs of research and development. Health expenditures in non-innovating countries will exclude the research and development costs."[26]

Many express alarm at rising health care spending, yet most would agree that higher incomes, longer life expectancy, and increased health care productivity are positive developments. Further, America's status as the world leader in developing new medical technologies, and foreigners coming to the United States to purchase medical care, are reasons to applaud additional health care spending. Though America's health care system engenders considerable waste, it is equally clear that many health care expenditures yield impressive returns.

Does the U.S. Spend More but Get Less?

The most important factor in evaluating how much a nation spends on medical care is whether it gets its money's worth. Critics of the U.S. health care system point out that despite large expenditures America does not compare well with other nations on such measures as life expectancy or infant mortality. For example, the Organization for Economic Cooperation and Development reports that the United States ranks below most other industrialized nations in infant mortality.[27]

Such measures, though, do not reflect the return America receives on its investment in health care. The cross-national comparisons on which such criticisms rely often are not direct comparisons, and often do not control for contributing factors unrelated to a nation's health care system. A significant portion of the gap in infant mortality rates is explained by what various nations consider a "live birth." The United States tends to include in its measure of live births extremely low–birth-weight infants whom other nations seem to exclude. One study noted that across 23 European countries "there are many indications of differences in recording and reporting live birth, fetal death, and infant death within the European region of the [World Health Organization]. Even when [standardized] recommendations are adopted as the legal definition, some countries have incomplete registration or reporting of events."[28]

Figure 1.5
PERCENT OF GDP SPENT ON HEALTH VS. LIFE EXPECTANCY AT
BIRTH FOR FEMALES (2002)

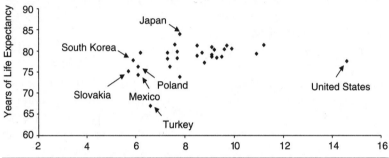

SOURCE: *OECD Health Data 2004*, 3rd Edition, Tables 1 and 10.

A more useful comparison of different health care systems is how well they cope with the same problem, such as infants of a given birth weight. Nicholas Eberstadt of the American Enterprise Institute notes that controlling for birth weight shows that the United States does a better job than other nations. "By comparison with other Western societies enjoying especially low rates of infant mortality, U.S. babies at any given birth weight appear to have unusually good chances of surviving the perinatal period, regardless of race," Eberstadt writes. "All other things being equal, this would seem to suggest that medical care for infants in the United States is actually rather better than in some other advanced industrial societies."[29]

Comparisons of life expectancy are also of limited use. There is little correlation among advanced nations between health care expenditures (whether absolute or as a share of GDP) and life expectancy (see Figure 1.5). The United States spends more than 14 percent of GDP on health care compared with South Korea's 6 percent, yet females born in the two countries have roughly the same life expectancy (79.8 years vs. 80.0 years). However, Poland, Slovakia, and Mexico each spend a share of GDP similar to South Korea's (6.1 percent, 5.7 percent, and 6.1 percent, respectively), yet have slightly lower life expectancies (78.8 years, 77.8 years, and 77.1 years, respectively). Turkey spends a slightly larger share of GDP (6.6 percent) on health care than South Korea, yet life expectancy for females is almost a decade less (70.9 years).

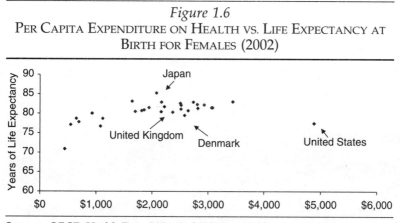

Figure 1.6
PER CAPITA EXPENDITURE ON HEALTH VS. LIFE EXPECTANCY AT
BIRTH FOR FEMALES (2002)

SOURCE: *OECD Health Data 2004*, 3rd Edition, Tables 1 and 10.

The actual amount spent per person on medical care would seem to be a more helpful predictor, but even this measure shows little correlation with life expectancy. Life expectancy for females born in Denmark is on par with those born in the United States (79.5 years vs. 79.8 years) even though per capita health care expenditures in Denmark are half what they are in the United States ($2,580 vs. $5,267) (see Figure 1.6). From this comparison, it would seem Americans could live longer by spending less. Yet consider Japan and the United Kingdom. Each spends roughly the same amount per capita on medical care ($2,077 vs. $2,160) yet life expectancy in Japan (85.2 years, the highest of any nation) is nearly five years more than in the U.K. (80.4 years).[30]

Clearly, there are variables other than health care spending that determine infant mortality rates and life expectancy, including genetic attributes, nutrition, and *how* nations spend their health care dollars. A better measure of a nation's health care system is how it performs when confronted with particular medical challenges. As noted earlier with regard to cancer patients and low-birth-weight infants, evidence exists that the United States outperforms other nations.

2. Real Problems

Costs

There is little misperception about the direction of health care costs. A 2004 survey found that while economists believe terrorism presents the greatest short-term risk to the economy, "In the longer run, the rising elderly population and related health care costs are the primary problems."[1] In another poll, more Americans expressed as much concern over health care as over terrorism and national security. The paramount concern is the cost of health insurance: "Americans are increasingly dissatisfied with the cost of health care."[2] For most of the past 18 years, the cost of employer-based health insurance has risen faster than workers' earnings and inflation. Year-to-year increases in health premiums routinely exceed 10 percentage points. In one survey, "Fifteen percent of employers said that they offset premium increases with smaller raises for their employees."[3] Health insurance has become increasingly burdensome for employers and consumers alike.

Perhaps more troublesome is the obligation of government health programs. Medicare is the federal program that provides health care subsidies to the elderly and disabled. Medicaid is a joint federal-state program of health care for the indigent. Each program places a large and growing burden on taxpayers. In 2006, the federal government spent a combined $554 billion on Medicare and Medicaid (not including the State Children's Health Insurance Program, a Medicaid offshoot). That is more than Congress spent on national defense ($520 billion). When state Medicaid spending is included, these two programs cost taxpayers an estimated $692 billion in 2006, more than one-quarter more than Social Security ($544 billion)[4] (see Figure 2.1). According to the Congressional Budget Office, Medicare spending will double from the 2007 levels in 10 years and federal Medicaid spending will nearly double in nine years.[5] If current trends continue, Medicare and Medicaid alone could consume 12 percent of GDP by 2030.[6]

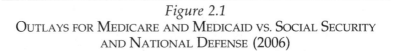

Figure 2.1
OUTLAYS FOR MEDICARE AND MEDICAID VS. SOCIAL SECURITY
AND NATIONAL DEFENSE (2006)

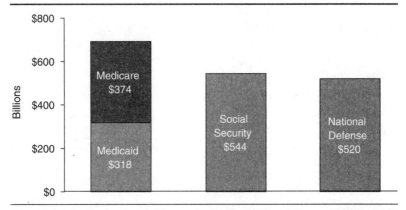

SOURCES: *The Budget and Economic Outlook: Fiscal Years 2008 to 2017* (Washington: Congressional Budget Office), pp. 50, 54, and author's calculations.

The danger posed by the growing burden of these two programs is difficult to overstate. The benefits promised to future Medicare beneficiaries under current law far exceed the capacity of existing revenue sources to meet those promises. If the federal government were to deposit funds in an interest-bearing account to cover all of Medicare's future deficits, the amount it would have to deposit in 2007 would be $74.6 *trillion.*[7] That amount is almost 70 percent larger than the combined GDPs of all the nations on earth, and about five times the size of the U.S. GDP and the amount required to cover Social Security's shortfalls.

Quality

As noted earlier, concerns about health care quality persist despite America's stature as a world leader in medical innovation. The quality of medical care delivered to American patients is often poor. Studies indicate that patients who could be helped by the most effective treatments do not receive them. One study in the *New England Journal of Medicine* found that adults receive, on average, the generally accepted standard of preventive, acute, and chronic care only about 55 percent of the time. The likelihood that patients would receive recommended care "varied substantially according to the particular medical condition, ranging from 78.7 percent of recommended care . . . for senile cataract to 10.5 percent of recommended care . . . for alcohol dependence."[8] Moreover, a lot of the health care that Americans consume seems to provide no improvements in health.

In particular, studies suggest that American patients are frequently harmed by errors made by medical professionals. Medical errors are a serious problem. The most commonly cited figures come from an Institute of Medicine study that suggests between 46,000 and 98,000 hospital patients die every year due to medical errors in the United States.[9] Another study estimated that medical errors are associated with over 192,000 preventable deaths annually, though only 81 percent of such deaths (about 155,000) were "potentially attributable" to medical error.[10] Studies suggest that many medical errors come from overworked interns[11] and overwhelmed pharmacists.[12] Thousands of preventable injuries and deaths may be due to unnecessary procedures.[13] America is not unique in this regard. A study of medical errors in Canada estimated that between 9,250 and 23,750 Canadian patients die every year following a medical error— the equivalent of 83,000 to 214,000 deaths in a country the size of the United States.[14] Patient surveys suggest similar numbers of medical errors in both countries.[15] Hospitals in a number of Canadian provinces have struggled with repeated incidences of deadly infections.[16]

Medical errors will continue to occur as long as and wherever humans practice medicine. When addressing the quality of medical care in the United States, policymakers should begin with a clear understanding of the extent of the problem and the role that competition plays in promoting quality.

Bureaucracy

Finally, the U.S. health care system seems awash in bureaucracy. One result is that many physicians are reporting less job satisfaction. The proportion of experienced physicians (ages 50–65) who report a decreasing level of satisfaction over the previous five years rose from 54 percent in 2000 to 76 percent in 2004.[17] At least part of this decline can be attributed to the bureaucracy involved in practicing medicine today. According to one survey, "Rather than declining income, threats to physicians' autonomy, to their ability to manage their day-to-day patient interactions and their time, and to their ability to provide high-quality care are most strongly associated with changes in satisfaction."[18]

PART II

MISDIAGNOSIS

3. How Not to Reform Health Care

With America's health care system presenting such symptoms, few would deny the need for reform. However, as many of the preceding criticisms indicate, the underlying condition is poorly understood. This misunderstanding has led to various prescriptions that would be far worse than the disease. As in the practice of medicine, the guiding philosophy of health policy should be, *First, do no harm.*

A "Right" to Health Care?

With millions of Americans priced out of the market for health insurance, some propose to have government recognize or declare a right to health care. Physicians for a National Health Program, a group that claims to represent more than 10,000 doctors and medical students, declares, "Access to comprehensive health care is a human right. It is the responsibility of society, through its government, to assure this right."[1] Sen. Edward M. Kennedy (D-Mass.) has remarked, "We have it in our power to make the fundamental human right to health care a reality for all Americans."[2] His colleague Sen. John F. Kerry (D-Mass.) has said, "I'm committed to universal health care coverage because, in America, health care is not a privilege, it's a right."[3]

Medical care can be as essential to survival as food. But does it follow that people have a right to medical care? Would recognizing a right to health care solve America's health care difficulties or add to them? We can answer these questions with a thought exercise. Suppose Congress and the states were to amend the U.S. Constitution by adding a legally enforceable right to health care.[4] Even if such a measure could win approval, the debate would not and could not end there.

The first difficulty would be to define the "right." What health care do Americans, by right, deserve? Do Americans have a right

33

to preventive care? What types of preventive care? Should mammograms be made available to all women, regardless of their likelihood of developing breast cancer? Health care researcher J. D. Kleinke notes that if government recommendations were followed, the number of Americans on drug regimens for hypertension, asthma, obesity, and high cholesterol would increase anywhere from 2- to 10-fold.[5] Spending on pharmaceuticals would explode. With the wide variety of medical tests and treatments that consumers may claim as their right, someone at some point must decide where the right to health care ends, lest the nation be bankrupted.[6] Those difficult questions helped derail a proposed constitutional right to health care in Massachusetts in 2007.[7]

Whoever has the power to make these decisions will exercise enormous power over who does and does not receive medical care. Who should have that power? In most nations that have tried to guarantee universal access to medical care, politicians allocate specified funds to local bureaucracies, which in turn decide how medical care will be rationed. This is typically achieved by making even seriously ill patients wait for care.[8]

A second and related difficulty is the question of who pays. A right to health care by definition would not be conditioned on one's ability to pay. Enforcing the right would require increasing taxes in proportion to how generously one defines the "right."

A third difficulty is the incentives such a system creates. Patients would have little reason to constrain their consumption because additional consumption would cost them little. Higher tax rates would discourage work and productivity, yielding less economic growth and wealth. Pushing down the compensation of medical professionals would discourage many (and many of the brightest) candidates from entering the field of medicine. Divorcing their compensation from the satisfaction of their patients would reduce the quality of care. Since innovations that increase medical productivity also increase spending, policymakers would discourage innovation because every new discovery puts them in the uncomfortable position of either increasing taxes or saying "no" to patients. The paradox of a "right to health care" is that it discourages the very activities that help deliver on that "right."

A final difficulty is how to deliver the medical care to which all are now entitled. Declaring health care to be a right does nothing to solve the problem of getting the right resources to the right place at the right time. Where are doctors most needed? Where will we place hospitals? Who will produce surgical tools? How much will they be paid? These decisions must be made through the political process. Not only has the political process proven slow and imprecise at meeting shifting needs, but those with political power would enjoy a greater "right" to health care than others by virtue of their ability to affect the allocation of health resources. That has largely been the experience of countries that have tried to enforce a right to health care.[9]

If comprehensive health care were a human right, it would have to be for citizens of other nations as well. Americans could not have a greater right to medical care as a result of having more wealth than citizens of India or Haiti. If all Indians and Haitians have a right to the same quality care as Americans, how should that care be financed?

Fundamentally, creating a legal "right" to health care is incompatible with the idea of individual rights. People cannot legitimately claim a right to something if that claim infringes on the rights of another. Smith's right to free speech takes nothing away from Jones. The only obligation Jones owes to Smith is not to interfere with Smith's exercise of her rights. The same is not true of a right to health care, which would turn the concept of rights from a shield into a sword by imposing an obligation on Jones to provide health care to Smith.

The underlying goal of creating a legal right to health care is to provide medical care to the greatest number possible. The fact that this approach would reduce the amount of medical care available to most or all Americans suggests that we should look for other ways of achieving this goal.

Government-Run Health Care

Whether or not government creates a legal right to health care, it could still manage and fund America's health care system, as is done in Canada, Europe, and elsewhere. Such proposals go by the names *single-payer, universal coverage, national health insurance,* or *national health care.* The details of these proposals vary, but in general they would finance the provision of health care through higher taxes. Government—whether the federal or a state government—would pay for all health care services, with reduced or no direct charges to patients. Private insurance could be restricted to services not covered by the government. Government would set an overall health care budget and reimbursement levels. Nobel laureate economist Milton Friedman notes that this idea "has great political appeal. It promises to provide quality health care to all, regardless of income, religion, race, or initial state of health."[10] But as Friedman and others have observed, the idea does not live up to the promise.

A government-run health care system would come at enormous cost to American taxpayers. One proposal championed by Representative and former Democratic presidential candidate Dennis Kucinich was estimated to cost as much as $6 trillion over 10 years.[11] Supporters argue that some of this cost would be offset by savings from reduced administrative costs and insurance company profits. However, research suggests that government provision of health care leads to higher administrative costs. Patricia Danzon has estimated that administrative costs under Canada's single-payer health care system equal more than 45 percent of claims, while the figure for private health insurance in the United States is less than 8 percent of claims. She writes, "The rough empirical evidence tends to confirm that overhead costs in Canada, adjusted to include some of the most significant hidden costs, are indeed higher than they are under private insurance in the United States."[12] On the one hand, supporters of national health insurance also predict savings from preventive care that the uninsured currently do not receive. On the other hand, most cost estimates do not include the increased demand that would follow the reduction or elimination of copayments and deductibles.

Americans would receive little return on such an investment. Shortages are characteristic of all national health care systems, and governments typically deal with those shortages by forcing patients to wait for treatment. At any given time, one million Britons are waiting to be admitted to their National Health Service hospitals, and shortages force the NHS to cancel some 100,000 operations per year.[13] Ninety thousand New Zealanders are in the same boat.[14] In Sweden's public hospitals, the average wait for heart surgery is 15 to 25 weeks. The average wait for hip replacement surgery is over a year.[15] (Waits in the United States are typically much shorter.[16])

More than 815,000 Canadians are currently waiting for medical care. One-half of Canadian patients referred to a specialist by a general practitioner wait longer than 8.4 weeks to see the specialist. Of the patients who go on to receive treatment, half wait longer than 9.5 *additional* weeks before being treated. Over half of all Canadian cancer patients wait longer for treatment than Canadian oncologists consider "clinically reasonable." On average, Canadian oncologists recommend a wait of no more than 3.4 weeks for radiation treatment, yet half of those patients wait at least 6.0 weeks. Half of all hip-replacement patients in British Columbia wait more than 22 weeks for the procedure. At the current rate it would take 65.8 weeks to treat all the hip-replacement patients in the province.[17]

Rationing by waiting imposes costs in terms of lives and health. In response to budgetary pressures, Britain has cut back on dialysis capacity to the point where the NHS can meet less than 82 percent of the need. Half of those waiting for dialysis in Britain suffer limitations on their ability to work or perform other daily activities. One-third report their health deteriorates while waiting. One out of seven claim to suffer significant pain as they wait.[18] In just one year, the Canadian province of Ontario removed more than 120 coronary bypass surgery candidates from its waiting list because they had grown too sick to benefit from the procedure.[19]

Countries with national health care systems also lag far behind the United States in the availability of modern medical technology. Even though Canada is fifth among advanced nations in the share of its economy it devotes to health care, it ranks in the bottom third of nations when it comes to access to medical technology.[20] Relative to population size, the United States has more than three times as many MRI scanners,[21] nearly four times as many lithotriptors,[22] and 65 percent more CT scanners than Canada.[23] Hospitals in Washington and Oregon are four times as likely to have cardiac catheterization facilities as similar hospitals across the border in British Columbia.[24]

Whatever its powers, government cannot repeal the laws of economics. When individuals perceive health care to be free, the quantity demanded increases. Faced with the choice of bankrupting their economy to pay for the virtually unlimited demand, or reducing the amount of health care provided, these countries opt for the latter.

Even with rationing, however, government-run health care systems do a poor job of controlling the rising cost of health care. When such factors as population growth, general inflation, exchange rates, growth in elderly populations, investment in research and development, and rates of crime, poverty, AIDS, and teen pregnancy are taken into account, Canadian health spending is much closer to that of the United States, and actually rose faster over much of the 1970s and 1980s.[25]

Universal health care is not free. Citizens of countries with national health care systems pay a heavy price in taxes. Canada's government-run health care system is one of the major reasons why the average Canadian family pays 47 percent of its income in taxes.[26]

"Managed Competition"

One step removed from government management of the health care marketplace is the concept of "managed competition." That idea would leave the provision of health care in private hands, but would create an artificial marketplace run under strict government control. Managed competition saw its fullest rendering in the failed Clinton health care plan.

The basic concept of managed competition is for employers and individuals to join so-called cooperatives that negotiate with private insurers offering a government-prescribed minimum set of benefits. Individuals choose among plans offered by their purchasing cooperative, with employers paying most of the premium. The premiums are priced the same for everyone in the plan, regardless of health status. Cooperatives serve not only to negotiate prices but also to gather relevant information for consumers about each available option.[27]

Managed competition actually exists in practice today, primarily among government employers and universities. The largest and best known model is the Federal Employees Health Benefits Program, which covers roughly nine million federal employees, retirees, and their dependents. The FEHBP exemplifies four basic features of managed competition. First, federal employees in most places can choose from among 8 to 12 competing health insurance plans. Second, the government contributes a fixed amount that can be as much as 75 percent of each employee's premium. Third, the employee pays the extra cost of more expensive plans. Fourth, the plans must charge all customers in a community the same amount, regardless of health risk.[28]

Another example of managed competition can be found in the Connector, a key part of the reforms enacted in Massachusetts in 2006 by then-governor Mitt Romney (R). The Massachusetts Health

Care Connector combines the state's small group and individual markets under a single unified set of regulations.[29] Supporters such as the Heritage Foundation consider the Connector to be the single most important change made by the legislation, calling it "the cornerstone of the new plan" and "a major innovation and a model for other states."[30]

The Connector is not an insurer, but rather a government bureaucracy that functions as a clearinghouse—a sort of wholesaler or middleman—matching customers with insurers and insurance products. It also allows small businesses and individuals to pool their resources to take advantage of the economies of scale available to large group plans.

Although the Connector does not technically regulate insurance, it has wide-ranging authority to determine what insurance products it will offer. For example, the maximum deductible allowed is $2,700 for an individual and $5,450 for a family. While this conforms to current rules regarding health savings accounts, it locks in those rules at a time when HSAs need to be made more flexible. (See Chapter 5.) Moreover, individuals choosing a high-deductible policy *must* combine it with an HSA. Health plans sold within the Connector must comply with the state's mandated benefits (with one exception noted later). They must also comply with the state's community-rating requirements and other restrictions designed to limit the ability of insurers to charge premiums according to risk.[31]

Beyond these restrictions, the Connector board is authorized to offer a "Connector seal of approval" to products that provide "high quality and good value." The Connector board itself is left to define what constitutes high quality and a good value. Significantly, however, that phrase frequently appears in legislation to describe plans that contain state-mandated benefits. The Connector may choose to allow products that do not receive its seal of approval, but it is not required to do so. As a result, the Connector effectively becomes a regulatory body, picking winners and losers from among insurance plans offered in the state.

No actual prohibition exists on selling small group or individual insurance outside the Connector. However, because Governor Romney's reform package makes subsidies and tax advantages available only within the Connector, and because of its competitive advantage in terms of pooling risk, the Connector eventually will squeeze out

---

Figure 3.1

ANNUAL PERCENTAGE INCREASE IN HEALTH INSURANCE PREMIUMS

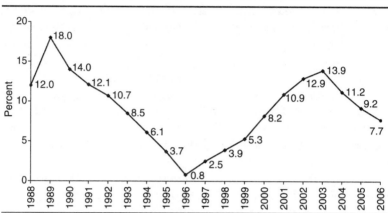

SOURCES: Kaiser/HRET: 1999–2006; KPMG Survey of Employer-Sponsored Health Benefits: 1993, 1996; The Health Association of America: 1988–1990.

any outside market. In the end, it would become a monopsony purchaser of health insurance.

Despite the problems with the Connector approach, several states are reportedly considering some variation of a Massachusetts-style Connector, including Iowa, Kansas, Louisiana, Maryland, Michigan, Texas, and Washington.

Managed competition is meant to spur competition between health plans, yet competition takes place on a very constrained basis. For example, health plans are not allowed to adjust their premiums on the basis of age, sex, or in many cases any risk factors. Plans can compete on the basis of services offered, but only on the margins, since all plans are required to offer the same package of core benefits. There is some limited price competition, but since plans cannot reduce costs by managing risks or through benefit design, even that is marginal. This is particularly problematic since an inability to price according to risk typically results in the overprovision of care to the healthy and the underprovision to the sick.

Managed competition relies heavily on managed care. However, managed care's record on controlling costs is mixed. As Figure 3.1 shows, when managed care truly began to penetrate the health care marketplace in the mid-1990s, health insurance premium growth did indeed slow down. Although many factors undoubtedly contributed, evidence exists that managed care succeeded in squeezing some waste and excess usage from the system. However, once the initial savings were achieved, health care costs began to rise again at about the previous rate. This is in part because resistance to restrictive cost-cutting measures forced managed care providers to loosen the spending reins, and in part because managed care did not resolve the perverse incentives that drive health care spending in the United States.

University of Chicago law professor Richard Epstein has noted that managed competition "is not so much a coherent government plan as an oxymoron. It is possible to have either managed health care or competition in health care services. It is not possible to have both simultaneously."[32] Even advocates agree that, in the words of one of its originators, Alain Enthoven, "Managed competition is not a free market."[33] In many ways, managed competition simply builds a layer of government control on top of all the worst features of the current system.

Employer Mandates

Another proposal would seek to make health care more accessible by requiring employers to provide health coverage to their workers. Such laws are called "employer mandates" and may require employers to provide health coverage to some or all workers, or give employers the option of paying taxes to a government program that does so. In 1974, Hawaii became the only state to implement an employer mandate.

The drawbacks of employer mandates outweigh any benefits. The amount of compensation each worker receives is a function of her productivity. Mandating an increase in a worker's compensation (through the provision of health insurance) increases the employer's operating costs, but does nothing to increase the worker's productivity. Employers therefore must find ways to offset the added costs imposed by the mandate. Their options include raising prices (which is unlikely in a competitive market), lowering wages, reducing wage increases, reducing health benefits (e.g., drug coverage, retiree health benefits), reducing other benefits (e.g., pensions), instituting layoffs, initiating automation, reducing hiring, hiring ineligible workers, outsourcing, and refusing to comply with the law. Noncompliance with Hawaii's mandate has been significant.[34]

In a 2004 statewide referendum, Californians rejected an employer mandate. The proposed law would have required employers either to provide coverage for their employees and their employees' families,[35] or to pay additional taxes to fund their workers' coverage through a government program. Studies of the proposed "pay or play" law suggested its cost would have been substantial. One estimated the law would have reduced the after-tax income of individuals earning $31,000 by 7 percent, while families earning that amount would have seen their after-tax income reduced 17 percent. Since employers cannot reduce compensation for workers at or near the minimum wage, as many as 38–45 percent of targeted workers would have lost their jobs rather than gain health insurance. Many affected firms would have raised prices, while others would have resorted to outsourcing or to hiring workers for fewer hours (making them ineligible).[36] Another study estimated the law would have cost as much as $13.2 billion, with only $4.4 billion going toward coverage for previously uninsured workers, and would have eliminated more than 218,000 jobs.[37]

Given the resulting job losses and other effects, it is unlikely that employer mandates can achieve their primary objective of expanding health coverage. What little study has been dedicated to Hawaii's law suggests that "the Hawaiian mandate did relatively little in extending insurance to the uninsured" and that Hawaii's high levels of health coverage relative to other states can be explained by population characteristics.[38] One study estimated that many California workers would avoid jobs that offer health insurance rather than accept lower wages, thereby *decreasing* the number of workers with health coverage.[39]

Nonetheless, employer mandates enjoy sporadic interest, in part because they allow government to tax consumers by hiding the burden in lower wages or reduced employment opportunities. Mandates also enjoy support among employers who already offer health benefits and can gain a competitive advantage by requiring their competitors who do not offer coverage to take on that added cost.[40]

For example, several states have considered health insurance mandates targeted at Wal-Mart. Maryland passed legislation in 2005 that would have required Wal-Mart to spend at least 8 percent of its payroll on health benefits or to pay an equivalent amount into the state's health program for the poor.[41] The courts ultimately struck down the legislation as a violation of federal law.[42]

In a surprising turn, California Gov. Arnold Schwarzenegger (R) proposed in 2007 to require all businesses with 10 or more employees to offer health insurance or to contribute 4 percent of their payroll to a state fund that would provide coverage to the uninsured.[43] Schwarzenegger made this proposal despite the fact that California voters had rejected a similar pay-or-play mandate in a 2004 statewide referendum.

A 2004 survey published in the journal *Health Affairs* found large majorities of workers supportive of an employer mandate. However, nationwide 56 percent believed an employer mandate would either reduce their wages or increase unemployment, and 51 percent of workers in California believed it.[44]

Individual Mandates

One of the most talked about approaches to universal coverage is a legal requirement that every American obtain adequate private health insurance coverage. Such a requirement is also known as an individual mandate. Those who don't receive such coverage through their employer or some other group would be required to purchase coverage on their own. Those who fail to do so would be subject to fines or other penalties.[45]

An individual mandate represents an unprecedented expansion of government power and interference in the economy. As the Congressional Budget Office noted when the idea was first raised in 1994, "The government has never required people to buy any good or service as a condition of lawful residence in the United States."[46] On a practical level, such a mandate is likely to prove unenforceable. More important, an individual mandate will almost certainly lead to a cascading series of additional mandates and regulations resulting, ultimately, in ever-greater government interference in the health care sector.

In April 2006, Massachusetts became the first state in the nation to enact such a mandate.[47] The bipartisan legislation was based on a proposal that then-governor Mitt Romney (R) had pushed for nearly two years.

Advocates of a mandate liken health insurance to automobile insurance. If government can require drivers to purchase auto insurance in order to protect society from the costs imposed by uninsured drivers, they argue, then government should be able to do the same thing with health insurance. This analogy between auto and health insurance is imperfect, however. First, driving has long been recognized as a privilege, subject to all manner of regulatory requirements. Second, if one does not like the regulations, including an insurance mandate, one can choose not to drive. Because it is easier to forgo a car than one's own body, a health insurance mandate would not generally give people such a choice. Third, states require drivers to purchase auto insurance for the protection of *others*—not the driver. Most states do not mandate that drivers carry insurance to cover their own injuries or repair costs.

Mandated automobile insurance does, however, show how difficult it is to enforce such mandates. Forty-seven states have laws mandating that drivers purchase automobile liability insurance, yet roughly 14.5 percent of drivers in those states are nonetheless uninsured. In some states, such as California and Mississippi, the uninsured motorist rate runs as high as 25 percent.[48] In some areas of Los Angeles, the uninsured rate reaches an astounding 75 percent.[49] The three states without mandatory auto insurance have roughly the same share of uninsured drivers—15 percent—as states where auto insurance is mandatory. Despite penalties ranging from loss of license to fines of $5,000 to even the impounding of vehicles, millions of drivers ignore the mandate.[50] In fact, millions of Americans purchase "uninsured motorist" coverage precisely to protect themselves in the event they are hit by an uninsured driver. Interestingly, in spite of widespread auto insurance mandates, the percentage of uninsured drivers is roughly the same as the percentage of Americans without health insurance.[51]

One reason insurance mandates are difficult to enforce is the challenge of tracking compliance. Here the government's record does not inspire confidence. No federal agency invests as much time, money, and effort in tracking Americans as the Internal Revenue Service. Yet it consistently fails to track down millions of Americans who fail to file tax returns. Every 10 years a scandal arises when the Census Bureau cannot locate several million residents. The most commonly proposed solution is to require that Americans submit proof of insurance when they file their federal income taxes. But about 18 million low-income Americans are not required to file income taxes, usually because their incomes are too low.[52] Another 9 million Americans who are required to file tax returns nonetheless fail to do so.[53] Already, we have identified as many as 27 million Americans that would be missed by such a tracking system. Moreover, many of these nonfilers will be elderly, homeless, or mentally ill. Others will have changed their address, perhaps multiple times.

Even if the government were able to determine that someone had not purchased health insurance, what penalties should apply? Ideas have been suggested ranging from loss of driver's licenses to direct fines. In Massachusetts, during the program's first year, the penalty for failing to obtain insurance will be the loss of the individual's personal exemption for the state income tax. The following year, the real penalty kicks in, a fine equal to 50 percent of the cost of a standard insurance policy.

As Gene Steuerle of the Urban Institute has noted, the administrative and enforcement costs of collecting the penalty would be enormous.[54] The Internal Revenue Service, for example, relies largely on voluntary compliance backed up by a slow and cumbersome legal process to collect taxes. And it does not require those with very small amounts of income to file. Even so, millions of Americans cheat or fail to file. Collecting a penalty for failure to insure would be much more difficult. "The [IRS] is simply incapable of going to millions of households, many of modest means, and collecting significant penalties at the end of the year," Steuerle writes.[55]

While an individual mandate is unlikely to achieve universal coverage or significantly reduce health care costs, it crosses an important line. An individual mandate accepts the principle that it is the state's responsibility to ensure that every American has health insurance. In doing so, it opens the door to widespread regulation of the health care industry and political interference in personal health care decisions. The result will be a slow but steady spiral downward toward a government-run health care system.

For example, in order to implement an insurance mandate, legislators and administrators will have to define what level of coverage fulfills that mandate. That guarantees that certain groups will try to influence the definition of "acceptable" coverage in a way that serves their special interests. Various health care providers will

45

demand that coverage of their particular services be included in the standard benefits package. Groups interested in particular diseases will do the same. The general public will either be unaware of such special interest lobbying or will consider each tiny increase in premiums to be too small to resist.

In Massachusetts, Governor Romney originally proposed making available a low-cost, no-frills policy that would make it easier for residents to comply with the individual mandate. However, by the time the legislature finished with the bill, residents were required to purchase insurance that included all the state's mandated benefits.[56]

As more benefits were added, the cost of the mandate would increase. That would place legislators in a very difficult position. If they increased subsidies to keep pace with the rising cost of the mandate, the cost of the program would explode. However, if they held subsidies steady, the increased cost would be borne by consumers, who would have no choice but to continue purchasing the ever more expensive insurance. Since the consumers would have little or no leverage over insurers (they can no longer refuse to buy their products), they could eventually be expected to turn to the government for subsidies.

Attempts to scale back benefits would certainly meet political opposition from powerful constituencies and complaints about "cuts." The only other alternative would be for the government to intervene directly by capping premiums. Insurers unable to charge more for an increasingly expensive product can be expected to trim costs by cutting back on their reimbursement rates to hospitals and physicians. The result ultimately will be covert rationing of health care services.

An individual mandate is akin to the first in a series of dominoes. "If you want to go down the road of an individual mandate, it's necessary to reform the entire health insurance system to make sure healthy people can get affordable coverage and sick people are not priced out of the market," says Gail Shearer of Consumers Union.[57]

The Massachusetts Health Care Connector is taking just those steps: subsidizing people here, taxing people there, using all its regulatory powers as best it can. Yet in 2007, the Connector board was forced to admit that even with an individual mandate it could not cover all of Massachusetts's uninsured. The board voted unanimously to exempt 20 percent of the uninsured from the individual

Figure 3.2
SHIFTING MODES OF FINANCING HEALTH CARE, 1965–2001

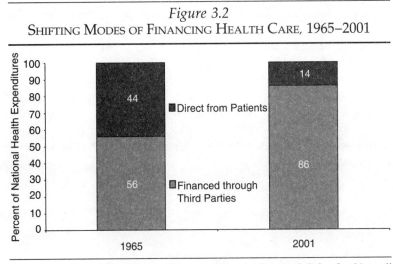

SOURCE: "National Health Care Source of Funds, Selected Calendar Years," 2003 Data Compendium, Centers for Medicare & Medicaid Services, November 2003.

mandate.[58] Along the way, however, the individual mandate vastly increased government control over Massachusetts residents' health care decisions.

Thinking Outside the Box

These and many other health care reform proposals operate from a background assumption that someone other than the consumer should control the consumer's health care dollars. That assumption is grounded in the fact that for generations more and more of America's health care bills have been financed through employers and government (see Figure 3.2). Consider that, in 2007, the average family of four paid roughly $14,000 in taxes to fund government health programs.[59] If the family had their own coverage, it cost them another $11,000 on average.[60] *Yet the family controlled none of that $25,000.* The government controlled the first portion, and their employer controlled the second. The idea that this is a natural state of affairs pervades discussions of health policy in the United States to the point where few even recognize they have adopted this article of faith.

This explains why the above-mentioned proposals and many others make "expanding coverage" a primary object. In a culture that expects a bureaucracy to finance nearly all medical care, lack of total coverage may be seen as the equivalent of lacking health care. Expanding coverage—or even achieving universal coverage—becomes the logical imperative. Few health care proposals think outside this box. As Chapter 4 discusses, health insurance coverage has its place. However, the idea that the object of health policy is to ensure universal coverage is an article of faith that must be reevaluated.

PART III

UNDERLYING DISEASES, STRONG MEDICINE

4. Too Much of a Good Thing Can Be Very Bad

What can policymakers do to make health care of ever-increasing quality available to an ever-increasing number of consumers? The answer begins with an accurate diagnosis of the problem. As discussed in the Introduction, producers in an open market must compete to meet consumers' needs at the lowest possible cost. Consumers who must weigh different options against one another tend to focus on getting the highest value per dollar spent, and they reward producers who provide it. Consumers and efficient producers both gain. Inefficient ways of doing things are driven from the market. Competition constantly pushes producers to reduce prices and improve quality. However, this process does not describe America's health care sector.

Why does health care lack the vigorous competition that produces wonders in other sectors of the economy? As we survey the scene, we see that many of the necessary conditions of healthy competition have been disabled. On the consumer side, government promotes excessive levels of health coverage. On the producer side, it imposes excessive regulation, which dampens competition. In each instance, government usually has a stated goal of making health care more affordable, protecting consumers, or even increasing market competition. However, its interventions often produce the opposite effect. When it limits experimentation and learning in the marketplace, government inhibits the competitive discovery process and most often leaves consumers worse off.

The good news is that policymakers can restore choice and competition to health care. First, they should reduce and eventually eliminate policies that encourage or hinder particular ways of financing medical care or insurance. That will require both short-term and long-term strategies that build on the success of health savings accounts. Second, policymakers should enable greater competition in the health care sector. That requires removing regulations that restrict providers' freedom to innovate, and patients' freedom to choose how to care for their minds and bodies.

The Trouble with Too Much Health Coverage

Health insurance plays a crucial role in financing health care. But Americans rely on health coverage beyond its usefulness. Like auto, fire, and homeowner's insurance, health insurance is supposed to protect against unlikely but high-cost events. Ordinarily, it would not cover regular checkups for the same reason that auto insurance does not cover oil changes: such expenses are neither unlikely nor high-cost. It is easier to pay for smaller, predictable expenses directly rather than through insurance. Of course, there is no reason why someone should not be able to purchase coverage for regular checkups—as long as she is willing to pay the added cost.

Health insurance works differently in the United States. Rather than have consumers evaluate the costs and benefits of different types of coverage, government actively hides the full cost of coverage from consumers. As a result, consumers demand more generous coverage, and much of the care covered by that health "insurance" is care that they otherwise would purchase directly. There are two main ways government hides from consumers the cost of their health coverage. First, the federal and state governments grant special tax treatment to employer-provided health insurance. As a result, most Americans obtain health coverage through an employer. That hides the cost of coverage because employers pay a portion or all of the premiums. (It also encourages more generous coverage because it exempts from taxation any medical care covered by an employer's health plan.) Second, government provides health coverage to tens of millions Americans through government programs. These programs hide the cost of coverage from the beneficiaries by passing the cost on to taxpayers. The cumulative result is that roughly 86 cents of every dollar spent on medical care in the United States today is financed through a third party (see Figure 4.1).[1] Government itself finances nearly half of all medical expenditures. In fact, the United States finances a greater share of its health care bills through third-party bureaucracies than 17 other advanced countries, including Canada (see Figure 4.2). By this admittedly crude measure, America's health care system is more socialized than many others.

Figure 4.1
PERSONAL HEALTH CARE SPENDING: DIRECT PAYMENT
VS. THIRD-PARTY PAYMENT (2002)

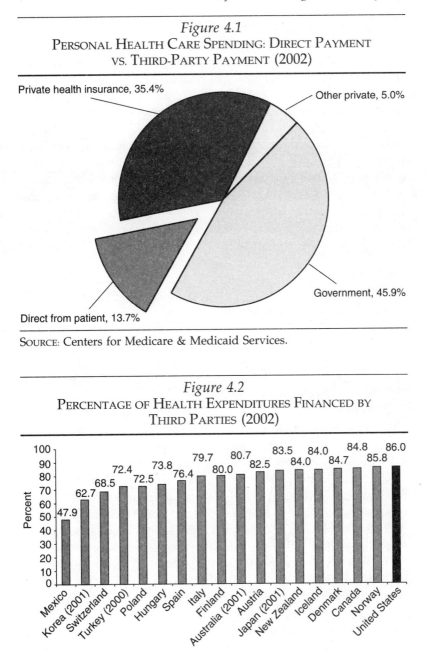

Private health insurance, 35.4%

Other private, 5.0%

Government, 45.9%

Direct from patient, 13.7%

SOURCE: Centers for Medicare & Medicaid Services.

Figure 4.2
PERCENTAGE OF HEALTH EXPENDITURES FINANCED BY
THIRD PARTIES (2002)

SOURCE: *OECD Health Data 2004.*

53

This overreliance on health coverage has far-reaching consequences. When patients enter the medical marketplace with excess coverage, they have less need to weigh the benefits of health care against the costs. They end up utilizing care that provides little value. Since patients are not very particular about costs and benefits, neither are providers. They have less incentive to focus on innovative ways of meeting patients' needs or to furnish information about prices and quality. Costs cannot help but rise in such a market. With insurers, employers, and government exercising more control over consumers' health care dollars, consumer choice inevitably suffers as well. All told, America's overreliance on health coverage reduces competition, increases costs, and decreases quality. What follows is a discussion of the problems created by this overreliance on health coverage, and how to reduce it.

Creating Conflict

Most fundamentally, America's overreliance on health coverage creates unnecessary conflict. In most markets, the interests of consumers, producers, and payers are well-aligned because the consumer and the payer are the same person. Producers get paid when they give consumers what consumers want. The lines of authority and accountability are clear. When the consumer and the payer are not the same person, however, it creates conflict between all three parties.

To some extent, this type of conflict is inevitable in health care. Many medical expenses are beyond most patients' ability to pay, so it makes sense for insurers to pay on their behalf. Any resulting conflict would normally be mitigated through deductibles and copayments. Coverage may begin only after patients have paid a certain dollar amount of care themselves, that is, after they meet their deductibles. Beyond that, the insurers may require the patients to pay a portion of the covered expenses, that is, a copayment. Deductibles and copayments give the patients an interest in eliminating wasteful expenditures and utilizing only medical care that they expect will provide value. These cost-sharing measures realign the interests of patients, payers, and providers. Having patients choose the terms of their health insurance in advance further harmonizes the parties' interests. This allows insurers to convey the costs of different ways of dealing with the problems of third-party payment (i.e., different deductibles, copayments, and other features) and requires consumers to weigh those costs.

When government hides the full cost of coverage from consumers, however, it makes the problem of conflicting interests worse. Lower deductibles make health insurance more expensive. Hiding the cost of lower deductibles—by passing the costs on to taxpayers or making it appear that one's employer is footing the bill—encourages lower deductibles, which creates conflict over low-cost medical expenses. Copayments likewise make coverage less expensive. Hiding the cost of eliminating copayments encourages people to eliminate copayments, and creates conflict over higher cost items.

One result is unnecessary conflict between patients and payers. Since patients pay an average of only 14 cents for each dollar of care, they utilize more care than they would if they had to shoulder more of the cost. The added utilization imposes costs on the people who ultimately pay for the other 86 percent—workers and taxpayers. They perceive no benefit from a stranger's overuse of the health care system. Through their agents (insurers, employers, and governments), they push back by refusing to pay for care that patients want. Excessive coverage also creates conflict between patients and payers by encouraging "moral hazard." By reducing the (apparent) costs to consumers of risky behaviors (e.g., obesity, smoking, reckless driving), it encourages consumers to do less than they otherwise would to safeguard their health.

Encouraging excessive coverage also creates conflict between payers and providers. Providers often see the payers' coverage decisions as an intrusion on the doctor-patient relationship and an affront to their professional judgment. One result is that providers (and presumably patients) often deceive payers to obtain coverage. Researchers from Yale University and Beth Israel Deaconess Medical Center in Boston found that 39 to 50 percent of physicians have manipulated third-party reimbursement rules to secure coverage of a particular treatment for a patient (and payment for themselves) (see Figure 4.3). Up to 70 percent of physicians said they would be willing to do so under certain circumstances.[2] The researchers wrote:

> Tactics reported by physicians have included exaggerating the severity of the patient's condition, changing the patient's diagnosis for billing, or reporting signs or symptoms that the patient did not have. Deceptions may involve brief changes in

Figure 4.3
PERCENTAGE OF PHYSICIANS WHO MANIPULATE THIRD-PARTY REIMBURSEMENT RULES

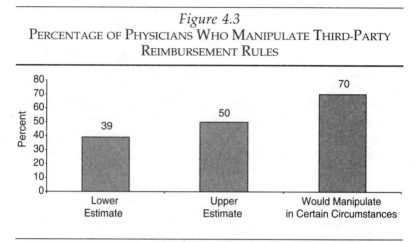

SOURCE: Sidney T. Bogardus Jr., David E. Geist, and Elizabeth H. Bradley, "Physicians' Interactions with Third-Party Payers: Is Deception Necessary?" *Archives of Internal Medicine*, Vol. 164, September 27, 2004, pp. 1841–44.

wording, as when physicians rule out cancer as the indication for a test rather than screening. Also, physicians may be willing to alter billing codes or to change elements of patient history (e.g., increasing the severity of a symptom or even creating nonexistent symptoms, such as claiming suicidal ideation to obtain a psychiatric referral) or results of physical examination (e.g., inventing findings such as breast lumps to obtain a referral for screening mammography).[3]

As one might imagine, physicians are increasingly likely to deceive third-party payers as reimbursement rules become more restrictive. Physicians who do so report that it is necessary to provide high-quality care and that their patients often ask them to deceive third-party bureaucracies. The researchers concluded that "deception is the symptom, not the problem," that "the use of deceptive tactics with third-party payers may be a signal that our health care financing system has a structural flaw," and that "we should be concerned about a system that places physicians in such a difficult position."[4]

In fact, America's overreliance on third-party payment results in exorbitant amounts of health care fraud. The *New York Times* recently reported that that state's Medicaid program "has become so huge, so complex, and so lightly policed that it is easily exploited." For example, one Brooklyn dentist billed the program for 991 procedures in a single day.[5] A federal oversight agency posits that fraud accounts for as much as 10 percent of all health expenditures in the United States,[6] which translates into some $226 billion in 2007.[7]

Encouraging excessive health coverage also creates unnecessary generational conflict. Elderly patients have high health expenses. Therefore, they benefit from generous government health programs. Younger workers have fewer health expenses, and benefit more from lower taxes. Hiding the cost of coverage for the elderly by shifting it to others creates conflict as different generations collide over tax rates and the generosity of government subsidies.

Vast sums of money are wasted on such conflict. Opposing patient, provider, and payer groups constantly apply pressure to government to influence the generosity of private and publicly provided health coverage. Health care interests spent more than $1 billion on political contributions and lobbying in the 2005–2006 election cycle.[8] Health care lobbying ranked second in terms of dollars spent in 2006.[9] Health professionals are the sixth-highest contributing profession to congressional campaigns.[10] The amount of money spent to influence government health policy may seem large, but it is a drop in the bucket compared with the amount of waste generated by America's overreliance on health coverage.

Overutilization, Wasted Resources, and Low-Quality Care

As noted earlier, excessive coverage encourages patients to utilize care without regard to its cost. Ordinarily, consumers spend $1,000 on an item only if they expect it to provide at least $1,000 of value. When spending someone else's money, however, their consumption patterns change. When it comes to health care, Americans demand care even if it provides less benefit than its cost. Since patients directly pay on average only 14 cents on the dollar for medical care, they tend to demand medical care that costs $1,000 even if it provides only $140 of value. Paul Ginsburg of the Center for Studying Health System Change and Len Nichols of the New America Foundation write, "When someone else pays . . . patients have little price sensitivity and almost no incentive to economize and make sure the expenditure is commensurate with the clinical value of the service."[11]

Newhouse and others involved in the RAND Health Insurance Experiment studied utilization among two groups of individuals.

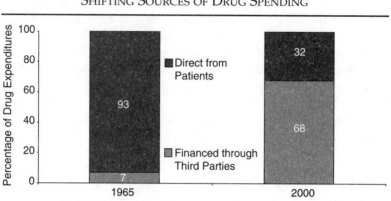

Figure 4.4
SHIFTING SOURCES OF DRUG SPENDING

SOURCE: Centers for Medicare & Medicaid Services, "Table 1.10—Spending for Prescription Drugs by Source of Funds, 1965–2000," An Overview of the U.S. Healthcare System: Two Decades of Change, 1980–2000.

The first group was given health coverage that made medical care effectively "free." The second group faced tradeoffs between medical care and other items for the first few thousand dollars of medical expenses. They found that families who faced tradeoffs between health and non-health items "reduced expenditure about 25 to 30 percent relative to a plan in which care was free to the family."[12] In other words, comprehensive coverage led patients to consume 43 percent more medical care than they otherwise would, despite the fact that it provided no measurable value.

A recent example of overutilization and wasted resources comes from a class of pain-relieving drugs called COX-2 inhibitors. As pharmaceuticals have become a more valuable tool for preventing and curing illness, health coverage has expanded to cover more drug costs. In 1965, 93 percent of spending on prescription drugs came directly from patients. By 2000, patients paid only 32 percent of their drug costs directly. Public and private coverage financed 68 percent (see Figure 4.4).[13] Because patients perceive the cost of an expensive drug to be less than it is, they often waste resources on expensive drugs when a cheaper alternative would have provided as much value. When COX-2 inhibitors became available, they offered no improvement in pain relief over existing, less expensive drugs.[14]

However, they were hailed for relieving pain without irritating the stomach as much as the alternatives.[15]

A study of Medicare patients with osteoarthritis found that those with the most drug coverage were twice as likely to use COX-2 inhibitors as those with the least drug coverage. This fact alone would not be troubling if the patients with more generous coverage needed the more expensive drug. But the study found they did not. In this group, patients who had little risk of adverse gastrointestinal reactions used the expensive COX-2 drugs as often as those at high risk, despite the availability of cheaper alternatives.[16] Another study found that more than 60 percent of prescriptions for COX-2 inhibitors were for patients at low or very low risk of gastrointestinal complications from alternative medications.[17]

These studies help explain how increasing productivity and enormous waste can be found side by side in America's health care sector. Many patients who utilize expensive new technologies experience no benefits. Imagine there are two equal-sized groups of patients— Groups A and B. Both groups take the same pain reliever, Drug A. Drug A completely relieves pain for Group A, but leaves Group B with substantial pain. Now imagine a technological advance—Drug B. This blockbuster drug costs twice as much as Drug A, but completely relieves pain for everybody. If *both* groups switch from Drug A to Drug B, everyone will be free from pain. However, 25 percent of the money spent on Drug B would be wasted because even though Drug B is a technological advance, Group A gains nothing from it. Group A was already experiencing zero pain, and therefore would double its expenditures for no additional benefit. America's health care sector produces enormous waste alongside productivity gains because our overreliance on health coverage gives patients every incentive to consume technological advances, even if the added expense does them no good.

The RAND Health Insurance Experiment confirms that people with excessive coverage utilize care that does nothing to improve health. Families who had to weigh the cost of the first few thousand dollars of medical expenses saw "little to no net adverse effect on health for the average person," compared with families with 100 percent coverage. "Indeed, restricted activity days fell."[18]

It may be impossible to estimate the total amount of waste in America's health care sector. However, it is almost certain to be in the hundreds of billions of dollars. Milton Friedman has estimated that without decades of government encouragement of excessive health coverage, per capita spending on medical care in 1997 would have been less than half the actual figure.[19]

Price and Quality Information

America's overreliance on coverage also reduces the availability of information on prices and quality. As noted, patients have less incentive to shop for low-cost, high-quality care. One survey found that only 12 percent of Americans do any research on the cost or quality of health care providers each year,[20] despite the fact that 20 percent of Americans use more than $1,800 of medical care each year.[21] Even among those with heart disease, 42 percent did no research on their medical condition or treatments.[22] A study in the *Journal of the American Medical Association* found that only 15 percent of patients even talk to their physician about out-of-pocket costs.[23]

Lack of Information for Patients

Providers have little incentive to generate and advertise price and quality information because patients tend not to use the information. Even when patients attempt to shop for value, they are stymied by a lack of information on prices and quality. The Federal Trade Commission (FTC) and Department of Justice (DOJ) observe, "The public has access to better information about the price and quality of automobiles than it does about most health care services."[24] Harvard University professor Regina Herzlinger quips, "there's virtually no price or quality information. You ever try to find out what the price is for a certain procedure? I mean you'd think, huh, probably easier to get some information out [of] the FBI."[25] Princeton's Uwe Reinhardt notes, "Only rarely, in a few locations, do American patients have access to even a rudimentary version of the information infrastructure on which the theory of [a] competitive market . . . rest[s]. The price[s] of health services are jealously guarded proprietary information."[26]

Even those prices that can be obtained do not allow patients to judge the social value of services, because the prices rarely reflect actual costs. Wide dissemination of useful price information puts providers at a disadvantage when negotiating reimbursements from third-party payers. Hospitals and other facilities typically negotiate payments from private health plans in secret, because revealing how much they charge one plan harms their ability to negotiate with other plans. University of California, Santa Barbara, health economist H. E. Frech notes:

> [P]eople will say . . . there's no price data in hospital markets. Well, in a sense, that's actually backwards. The problem is there are millions of prices. There's too many prices. [F]irst there are thousands of services that are individually priced on the fee-for-service side, and the definitions aren't even perfectly standardized. The second point is, a typical hospital will have at least tens and maybe hundreds of payers with different prices. [T]he prices [are] not only different, the very bases of the price, what gets priced, is different.[27]

Bureaucracies are slow to demand quality data and can use it to eliminate wasteful expenditures only with difficulty. In all, as Herzlinger notes, "Health care 'Zagats' falter because health insurers—rather than consumers themselves—do the shopping."[28]

Lack of Information for Providers

An overreliance on coverage also denies providers information that a functional marketplace would furnish. When consumers are spending their own money, each purchase transmits information about their preferences, enabling producers to respond by providing more of what consumers value. Greater demand for hybrid cars leads to higher prices, and higher prices tell producers to invest more in hybrid cars. But because patients are less quality- and cost-conscious in the medical marketplace, providers have less access to information about what products, services, and delivery systems patients value most.

When patients take less care to weigh the expected costs and benefits of medical care, it conceals information about patient preferences from providers. Instead, payments to providers are based on what is important to insurers, employers, and government. As the FTC and DOJ observe, "At present . . . most payments to providers have no connection with the quality of care provided."[29] Instead, "providers who deliver higher quality care are generally not directly rewarded for their superior performance." Worse, "providers who deliver lower quality care are generally not directly punished for their poorer performance and, worse still, may even be rewarded

61

with higher payments than providers who deliver higher quality care."[30]

It should come as little surprise, then, that in practice, patients often receive substandard or unnecessary care. As noted earlier, U.S. patients receive the generally accepted standard of care only about half of the time. And having health insurance does little to improve the quality of care that patients receive.[31]

Ginsburg and Nichols argue that the lack of price and quality information may fuel the overconsumption that results from excessive coverage. "The impact of low patient out-of-pocket costs—coupled with payment systems that encourage providers to deliver more services," they write, "is probably magnified by limited information about the effectiveness of many medical tests and procedures."[32]

Dampened Competition

Discouraging patients from shopping for value and distracting physicians from pursuing higher quality care at lower prices cannot help but stifle competition. Michael Porter and Elizabeth Teisberg write,

> The most fundamental and unrecognized problem in U.S. health care today is that competition operates at the wrong level. It takes place at the level of health plans, networks, and hospital groups. It should occur in the prevention, diagnosis, and treatment of individual health conditions or co-occurring conditions. It is at this level that true value is created—or destroyed—disease by disease and patient by patient. It is here where huge differences in cost and quality persist. And it is here where competition would drive improvements in efficiency and effectiveness, reduce errors, and spark innovation. Yet competition at the level of individual health conditions is all but absent.[33]

Even where health plans, networks, and hospital groups compete with one another, it is often for the business of institutions—employers, health plans, government—rather than individual consumers. And even where consumers have a choice of health plans, it hardly amounts to a competitive environment.

Sixty percent of Americans obtain health insurance through their employer.[34] More than half (53 percent) of workers offered employer-provided coverage have at most two options.[35] Even where multiple options exist, it hardly amounts to a competitive environment. Herzlinger writes,

> [E]ven when companies offer three or four options, precious little distinguishes them—most managed-care plans provide the same benefits, insure virtually identical levels of expenses, reimburse providers in similar ways for a limited array of traditional services, and last for only one year. In essence, managed care comes in just two flavors: plans that place constraints on access to physicians and hospitals for a lower price, and plans that offer readier access for a higher price.[36]

Undermining the Doctor-Patient Relationship

Most physicians now rely extensively on third-party payers. More than 95 percent of physicians accept Medicare patients.[37] In 2001, about 90 percent of physicians had at least one managed-care contract, and on average physicians received roughly 40 percent of their income from managed care. Only about a quarter of physicians practiced independently, compared with 41 percent in 1983.[38]

This trend has had a negative impact on the way physicians practice medicine and the doctor-patient relationship. Swiss medical ethicist Ernest Truffer argues that the increasing interjection of "gate keepers," "case managers," and other forms of bureaucracy between doctors and patients "amounts to a rejection of the *medical* ethic—which is to care for a patient according to his specific medical requirements—in favor of a *veterinary* ethic, which consists of caring for the sick animal not in accordance with its specific medical needs, but according to the requirements of its master and owner, the person responsible for paying any costs incurred."[39]

When doctors are paid a set amount per office visit, as they often are, it leads to less time to meet with patients, which can have an impact on effective diagnoses and treatment. After receiving a second opinion that corrected a serious misdiagnosis (which missed three blocked coronary arteries), author Jay Neugeboren observed,

> the way the health care system is now run [has] undermined the traditional doctor-patient relationship. Not only do doctors have less and less time to meet with us, but, given the vagaries of health insurance, the doctor we see one time may not be the same doctor we see the next time, and so we often remain strangers to one another ... [I]n the words of Dr.

> Bernard Lown, inventor of the defibrillator, listening to the patient and taking a careful history remains "the most effective, quickest and least costly way to get to the bottom of most medical problems."[40]

A growing movement among some physicians to reject third-party coverage attests to the impact it has had on the practice of medicine and the physician-patient relationship.[41]

Stop Stacking the Deck against Patients

The most important step policymakers can take to improve the quality and affordability of medical care and to reduce wasteful medical expenditures would be to stop stacking the deck against patients by encouraging Americans to overrely on health coverage. The FTC and DOJ counsel:

> Private payors, governments, and providers should experiment further with payment methods for aligning providers' incentives with consumers' interests in lower prices, quality improvements, and innovation. Payment methods that give incentives for providers to lower costs, improve quality, and innovate could be powerful forces for improving competition in health care markets.[42]

Eliminating or minimizing government encouragement of excessive coverage would fulfill this objective and more.

Reducing such incentives would realign the self-interest of patients, providers, and payers, and would free providers to focus on their patients' interest in lower costs, higher quality, and greater innovation. Former Medicare trustee Tom Saving and Andrew Rettenmaier of Texas A&M University write, "When consumers care what health care costs, suppliers will have to compete for consumer dollars and this competition will reduce the cost of care."[43] Reducing incentives for excessive coverage would also reduce wasteful expenditures.

Finally, it would generate information on price and quality. Patients' purchasing behavior would give producers the information they need to focus on the goods and services that patients value most highly. This would spur greater competition among producers, and encourage them in turn to generate and advertise the price and quality information that patients require. According to Porter and Teisberg, "Encouraging competition at the level of specific diseases or conditions will speed the development of the right kind of information."[44] The FTC notes that "competition can help address . . . information problems by giving market participants an incentive to deliver truthful and accurate information to consumers . . . Studies by the FTC's Bureau of Economics have confirmed that advertising provides a powerful tool to communicate information about health and wellness to consumers—and the information can change people's behavior."[45] More information and greater competition will further drive the market toward lower costs and higher quality.

Eliminating government encouragement of excessive health coverage will require both fundamental tax reform and reform of government health programs such as Medicare, Medicaid, and the veterans health system. The necessary tools may be different in different instances. In each case the object is the same: to allow patients to choose how their health care dollars are spent.

5. Tax Policy and Health Care

Since World War II, the federal government has maintained an uneven playing field in health insurance markets. During the war, employers offered health benefits as a way to attract workers without running afoul of wartime wage controls. The federal government treated such benefits as a business expense exempt from taxation.

Eventually written into law, the tax exemption of employer-provided health insurance has two principal effects. First, it lowers the cost of employer-provided health insurance (including any medical care financed through such "insurance") relative to other goods and services. On the one hand, at a tax rate of 50 percent, purchasing $1 of goods requires $2 of pretax earnings. On the other hand, the same amount of pretax earnings buys $2 of health coverage. This preferential tax treatment makes the price of health insurance and medical care appear much lower relative to other expenditures, and encourages workers to purchase more coverage and consume more care than they otherwise would.

The second effect is that most Americans get their health insurance through employers, and most of their medical bills are paid by employers or insurers. In 2003, an estimated 60.4 percent of Americans obtained health insurance through an employer.[1] Already encouraged to overconsume health care by distorted prices, workers are further insulated from the cost of their health care consumption because someone else is paying the bill.

Since the tax benefits applied only to health care financed through the employer's health plan, health "insurance" came to cover not only catastrophic episodes but routine expenses as well. In 2004, 50 percent of workers in preferred provider organizations (PPOs) faced an in-network deductible of less than $500, and another 30 percent had no deductible.[2] As of 2003, nearly three-fourths of workers with employment-based coverage faced only a $15 copayment or less to see a physician (see Figure 5.1). Seventeen percent faced no copayment.[3] Health "insurance" has expanded to cover routine care

Figure 5.1
WORKERS' COPAYMENTS FOR PHYSICIAN VISITS (2003)

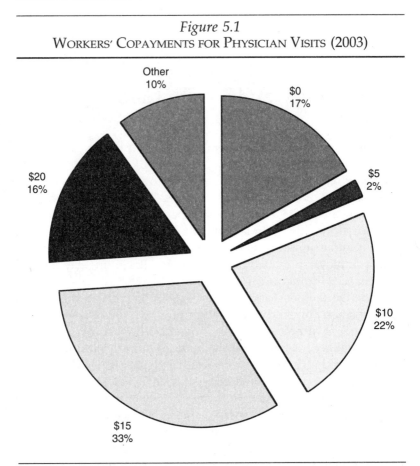

Other
10%

$0
17%

$5
2%

$20
16%

$10
22%

$15
33%

SOURCE: Kaiser/HRET Survey of Employer-Sponsored Health Benefits, 2003.

because financing these items through a third party brought tax benefits. Saving for one's routine medical expenses did not.

This uneven playing field has restricted consumer choice and competition, reduced patients' control over their health care decisions, increased the cost of health insurance and medical care, caused many to go without health insurance for extended periods (and many more for brief spells), discouraged saving, lowered wages, eliminated jobs, reduced consumers' health insurance choices, discriminated against those who cannot obtain employer-sponsored coverage, and left Americans poorer. In 2003, however, the federal government took the first step toward leveling this playing field by creating health savings accounts (HSAs). HSAs level the playing field somewhat between direct payment and third-party payment for health services. Congress should take further steps to level the playing field by enhancing and expanding HSAs, and ultimately enacting fundamental tax reform that removes the federal tax code's influence over consumers' health care decisions.

Effects of the Tax Exclusion

The cost of health care has placed a steadily rising burden on employers and workers. For over a decade, the cost of health insurance has risen faster than both workers' earnings and inflation. Health insurance premiums for a family of four increased by more than 10 percent in 9 of the past 16 years.[4] A study by Katherine Baicker and Amitabh Chandra of Dartmouth College estimates that a 10 percent increase in health premiums lowers wages by 2.3 percent, lowers a worker's likelihood of being employed, and lowers hours worked.[5] Another study estimates that rising health insurance premiums lead to a $1 reduction in health benefits for every $2 in reduced wages.[6]

From 2000 to 2006, private health insurance premiums increased by 86.5 percent—more than four times the rate of average earnings (19.6 percent).[7] As a result, by one measure the share of the population without health insurance grew by 3 percentage points between 1987 and 2005.[8] The percentage of nonelderly Americans receiving insurance through their employers declined from 68 percent in 2000 to 63 percent in 2005.[9]

Because employers see these higher costs in their budgets, they have attempted to constrain unnecessary spending with administrative controls that interfere with patients' medical decisions and how providers practice medicine. Employers have turned to managed care to control costs by restricting the number of providers and services eligible for coverage. In 1988, 27 percent of insured Americans were enrolled in some form of managed care plan. By 2004, that figure had risen to 95 percent.[10] As a result, more patients must comply with bureaucratic rules over how their own health care dollars may be spent. One survey found that the strongest predictor of dissatisfaction with a health plan, as measured by unwillingness to recommend the plan to others, is lack of choice with respect to providers.[11] In effect, managed care employs bureaucracies to constrain the consumption of patients who would constrain themselves if they were spending their own money. Managed care is a predictable outgrowth of America's overreliance on health insurance coverage.

Encouraging most Americans to purchase employer-provided health insurance has led to fewer choices both in the employer market and in the market for individual (as opposed to group) health insurance. As noted earlier, 53 percent of workers offered employer-provided coverage have at most two options. Nearly 90 percent of companies with fewer than 200 employees offer only a single health plan.[12] Consumers shopping in the individual health insurance market have their choices restricted by higher premiums[13] and the necessity of paying with after-tax dollars.

The rising cost of health benefits is considered a significant factor behind wage stagnation and the reluctance of employers to hire more full-time workers.[14] From 1989 to 2004, overall compensation rose by 12.7 percent, adjusted for inflation. But wages rose just 7.5 percent, while nonwage benefits increased 26.2 percent.[15] Industry sectors that are most likely to offer health insurance to employees and offer the most generous plans have suffered the biggest job losses in the past few years. Conversely, the greatest job growth has been in industries that offer few or less comprehensive health benefits.[16]

Unlike nearly every other type of insurance, health insurance in the United States is tied to employment. When workers leave their jobs, they also leave their health benefits behind. Thus the tax exclusion progressively decreases labor mobility and entrepreneurship by workers who fear losing health benefits. Studies have estimated that "job lock" reduces job mobility among married men by 22 percent and married women by 33 percent and is growing[17] (see Figure 5.2).

By encouraging overreliance on health coverage, the tax exclusion leads to moral hazard. It not only encourages riskier behaviors (smoking, overeating, inactivity), it also discourages prudent behaviors (saving for future medical expenses, exercise, preventive care) by creating the expectation that one's medical expenses are another's responsibility.

Finally, it leaves Americans substantially poorer. Harvard economist Martin Feldstein has estimated that the tax exclusion misallocates resources to health care that would have provided greater value if applied elsewhere. As a result, it cost Americans an estimated $126 billion in 2004.[18] This amounts to a hidden tax of nearly $1,000 per household.[19]

Figure 5.2
EMPLOYER-BASED HEALTH COVERAGE AND "JOB LOCK"

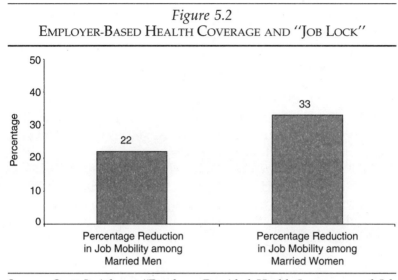

SOURCE: Scott J. Adams, "Employer-Provided Health Insurance and Job Change," *Contemporary Economic Policy*, Vol. 22, No. 3, July 2004, pp. 357–69.

Despite the damage the tax exclusion does by promoting health coverage well beyond the value it provides, it enjoys considerable support. Many workers and employers oppose removing the exclusion because doing so understandably *appears* to be a tax increase. Yet as Duke University professor Clark Havighurst notes, "a tax subsidy is insidious precisely because, in addition to being an off-budget public expenditure, it can misallocate huge amounts of society's resources, yet be entirely painless at the level of individual producers and consumers."[20] The fact that the exclusion's $126 billion hidden tax is hidden makes it no less real.

Health Care Reform Requires Tax Reform

If government imposes a tax, its purpose should be to raise revenue, not to encourage people to purchase health care versus other items, or to favor particular methods of financing health care. Ideally, tax policy would be neutral toward health expenditures and different methods of financing health care. However, repealing the current tax exclusion is politically infeasible and would be perceived as a tax increase as previously untaxed health expenditures would become subject to taxation.

To eliminate completely the differential tax treatment of health and nonhealth expenditures—and thus the tax code's bias toward excessive coverage—fundamental tax reform is necessary. A broad-based tax system that taxes health and nonhealth expenditures alike at a flat, low rate would accomplish this and be far preferable to the current federal income tax. Individuals would then make health care decisions according to what provides them the greatest value, not the greatest tax benefit. Health insurers and health care providers would have to compete aggressively for consumers, and the control that third parties currently wield over patients' medical decisions would disappear. As House Ways and Means Committee Chairman Bill Thomas (R-Calif.) has said, "Together we can solve the problem, or together we can continue to try to argue that . . . God created the employer deduction."[21]

Health Savings Accounts: Consumer-Directed Health Care

Fortunately, the federal government has taken a step toward reforming private health insurance through tax reform. In 2003, Congress and President Bush created HSAs, which extend the preferred tax treatment of employer-provided health insurance to personal, individually owned savings accounts that are dedicated for medical expenses. HSAs have the potential to bring important changes to both privately and publicly financed health care in the United States.

An HSA is much like a 401(k) dedicated for medical expenses. As with a 401(k), eligible individuals and their employers can make tax-free contributions. Earnings are also tax-free. Funds withdrawn before age 65 are generally taxed as income, plus a 10 percent penalty. After age 65, withdrawals are taxed as income with no penalty. However, in contrast to 401(k)s, *withdrawals for medical expenses are never taxed*. This is true before and after age 65. For this reason, HSAs have been described as "a 401(k) on steroids."

There are additional differences. To be eligible for an HSA, individuals must be covered by a qualified high-deductible health plan. In 2007, deductibles could be no lower than $1,100 for individuals and $2,200 for families. Deductibles could be no higher than $5,500 for individuals and $11,000 for families—which are also the limits on overall cost-sharing allowed with an HSA-qualified health plan.[22]

These plan design regulations effectively restrict HSA eligibility to those who have "qualified" coverage.

HSA contributions are limited to $2,850 for individuals and $5,650 for families. HSA holders between the ages of 55 and 65 may make additional "catch-up" contributions. The maximum amount for catch-up contributions is $800 in 2007. The figure increases by $100 per year until it reaches $1,000 in 2009.

HSAs are a milestone in health care policy. By reducing government encouragement of excessive private coverage, HSAs will restore much of the consumer sovereignty, product choice, and producer competition that have been eroded by government. HSAs reestablish the freedom to choose one's doctor, to own one's health insurance, and to self-insure for future medical needs without bureaucratic interference or being penalized by government. HSAs can help change the culture of health care in the United States by reorienting patients to shop for value and reorienting providers to enhance quality and contain costs. Although HSAs do not remove the differential tax treatment of medical expenditures, they do level the playing field between third-party coverage and self-insurance. Unlike other forms of health coverage, whatever patients do not spend from their HSAs, they keep in their accounts, which follow them from job to job.

In just 15 months, HSA enrollment reached over one million covered lives. By the end of 2004, more than 70 insurance companies had announced their intention to offer HSAs.[23] In November 2004, Kaiser Permanente, one of the nation's largest managed care organizations, announced it would offer an HSA because "our customers want to buy it."[24] BlueCross/Blue-Shield announced it would offer HSAs in 49 states and the District of Columbia by the first quarter of 2006.[25] Rather than list the name of every insurer offering an HSA product, *Health Market Survey* writes, "the easiest way to say it [is] *everybody* will be doing HSAs."[26] An estimated 4.5 million to 6 million Americans had HSA coverage by January 2007, and HSA enrollment was growing faster than that in other types of consumer-directed plans.[27] In a 2004 survey, a plurality of economists chose health savings accounts as the way to reform the U.S. health sector: "Forty-one percent of our panelists voted to institute health saving plans with a catastrophic insurance back-up." They also preferred them to a government-run health system by a ratio of more than two to one.[28]

HSAs have the potential to revolutionize much of the health care sector. However, their growth and success are hampered by unnecessary restrictions. In essence, these restrictions substitute the judgment of politicians for the preferences of individual consumers, and preserve much of what government does to encourage overreliance on third-party coverage. In practice, they limit the number of Americans who can open an HSA, the choices available to those interested in HSAs, and the ability of HSAs to contain health care costs.

The Next Step: Large HSAs

Whether HSAs will achieve robust growth may depend on whether Congress will enhance and expand HSAs into larger, more flexible accounts. Large HSAs would give workers full ownership of their health benefits and expand their freedom to control their medical decisions. Three changes are necessary:

(1) Increase HSA contribution limits to allow employers to deposit the full value of workers' health benefits directly into their HSAs.
(2) Eliminate the health insurance requirement for HSAs.
(3) Allow tax-free HSA withdrawals for all health insurance premiums.

Expanding HSAs in this way would all but eliminate government encouragement of excessive coverage and employer-directed health care. Whether deposited by employers or individuals, HSA funds would belong to individual consumers. They would control their health care dollars and decisions free of government encouragement of excessive coverage. Any bias toward employer-provided coverage would be eliminated as well. (However, employers would still have an incentive to make HSA deposits to avoid payroll as well as income taxes.)

Increase Contribution Limits

Current HSA rules continue to give workers a tax benefit only if they let their employers control their health coverage. Allowing workers to deposit the full amount of their health benefits into their HSAs would return that control to the workers themselves. Congress should set HSA contribution limits as high as the most that any employer and worker jointly contribute toward tax-free health benefits. For example, the Lewin Group estimates that more than 98 percent of singles receive $10,000 or less per year in untaxed health benefits. Ninety-eight percent of families receive $17,000 or less.[29] Capping HSA contribution limits in this range would have a number of benefits. It would give employers the flexibility to make their entire contribution toward workers' health benefits directly into the workers' HSAs. In turn, the workers would have the flexibility to use their HSAs to purchase health insurance from their employers or elsewhere. It would also impose a cap on the tax exclusion, an idea favored by many health care and tax experts. Unlike most proposals to do so, however, it would increase the workers' control over their earnings and their health care dollars.

Eliminate Insurance Requirement

Current law contains restrictions that limit both the appeal of HSAs to consumers and the ability of HSAs to contain health care costs. Americans are permitted to open an HSA only if they have a qualified health plan. In effect, this means that Congress grants the right to save tax-free for one's medical expenses only to those (1) who can afford to purchase health insurance and (2) who buy rigidly defined policies with restrictions on the number of deductibles (only one is permitted), the size of the deductible, and maximum amount of coinsurance. As noted, most Americans are not accustomed to health insurance with deductibles of $1,000 and higher. Many do not have sufficient savings to cover that kind of out-of-pocket exposure. That alone will deter many consumers from even considering an HSA.

However, lifting the insurance requirement would allow anyone to combine an HSA with their existing coverage, instantly making HSAs a feasible option for millions. In fact, lifting the insurance requirement would encourage more Americans to choose high-deductible insurance than do now. The opportunity to open an HSA will cause many consumers with low-deductible coverage to gravitate toward high-deductible coverage. As workers with low-deductible coverage accumulate savings, they would be able to cover more out-of-pocket costs. As a result, they likely would move toward higher deductibles to save money on their premiums. Allowing them to proceed gradually would entice more Americans to make the switch.

Lifting the insurance requirement would also give workers the option not to purchase health insurance at all, but accumulate savings in their HSA instead. Over time, these workers would also gravitate toward high-deductible health coverage. As those HSA holders see their balances grow, many eventually will purchase insurance to protect their savings from being wiped out by a catastrophic illness. Moreover, many HSA holders benefit by paying the rates that their insurer has negotiated with providers. Access to negotiated rates when paying out-of-pocket would further encourage uninsured HSA holders to obtain coverage.

One of the most frequent (and accurate) criticisms of existing HSAs is that while they can discourage wasteful spending on routine care, they may do little to reduce wasteful spending where restraint is needed most. Lifting the insurance requirement can remedy this. In a given year, more than 70 percent of all spending on medical care comes from the 10 percent of Americans who each consume more than $4,000 per year. Over half of all spending (56 percent) comes from the top 5 percent, who each consume more than $8,000 of care.[30] Yet the insurance requirement limits the ability of insurers to experiment with copayment structures that encourage patients to be prudent consumers when they require such levels of care.

In 2007, an individual could have a deductible of no less than $1,100 and a maximum out-of-pocket exposure of no more than $5,500. That means that after an HSA holder exceeds her deductible, there can be no more than $4,400 of copayments. Front-loading these allowable copayments (i.e., requiring relatively high copayments for relatively low-dollar expenses) reduces waste on care consumed closer to the deductible. However, it also leaves more high-dollar medical expenses exposed to the problems of third-party payment. Lifting the insurance requirement will enable insurers to find cost-sharing structures that make coverage more affordable while giving consumers the protection they want.

The most important reason to lift the insurance requirement is that it is the right thing to do. Government has no business telling consumers whether they should purchase health insurance or what type of insurance they should buy. Some consumers prefer lower deductibles and out-of-pocket exposure than HSAs currently allow, while some prefer higher deductibles and out-of-pocket exposure. HSAs are an attempt to remove government influence from consumers' decisions about health care and insurance. It perverts the principle underlying HSAs for government to require Americans to purchase any health insurance, much less a particular type of insurance, in order to be afforded the same opportunity to save for their medical expenses as other Americans. Allowing HSAs to be combined with any type of insurance will foster much more diversity and competition in health insurance markets, and greatly expand HSAs' appeal. In 2003, the House of Representatives passed legislation that would have expanded HSA eligibility to the uninsured as well as to those with more varied types of health insurance.[31] Congress should expand on that vote by lifting the insurance requirement altogether and allowing consumers to open a tax-preferred HSA regardless of their insurance status.

Deductibility of Individual Health Insurance Premiums

Since World War II, individuals have had to purchase health insurance with after-tax dollars, while employers could use pretax dollars. (Only recently has Congress allowed self-employed individuals to use pretax dollars.) This inequitable arrangement discriminates against the unemployed, those who do not receive health insurance on the job, and workers who do not want the coverage their employers offer. Moreover, it contributes to the problem of "job lock" discussed earlier.

Congress should correct this inequity by allowing individuals to purchase health insurance with HSA funds. This would allow all individuals, even those without employer-sponsored coverage, to purchase health insurance with pretax dollars. Allowing full deductibility of individually purchased insurance in this way would make coverage more affordable for millions and further level the playing field between employer-sponsored coverage and other types of insurance.

Large HSAs would give individuals full ownership of their health care dollars and greater choice of providers and insurers. Much like with 401(k)s, workers could decide how much to deposit into their HSAs and could vary their contributions from year to year. Workers could choose whatever type of health insurance they wished or they could forgo health insurance to build larger HSA balances and pay for health care expenses directly.

Large HSAs would also be far more equitable than the current exclusion. Today, high earners receive the largest tax benefits from the exclusion, while many low-income workers do not receive any benefit because their employers do not offer coverage. Large HSAs would allow all individuals to channel part of their wages to an HSA, and eliminate the disparities that result from the current exclusion. Even low-income workers who pay no income taxes would benefit from the exclusion of HSA deposits from payroll taxes.

Large HSAs would create more competitive health care and insurance markets. Providers and insurers would have to focus on the needs of individual consumers rather than the businesses they work for. Health care consumers would be more parsimonious when spending their own money, thus forcing producers to provide higher-quality, lower-cost services, and to provide better information to help patients make good decisions.

Large HSAs would also reduce administrative costs for employers. Employers would be able to maintain their current level of health benefits while eliminating the layers of bureaucracy required to administer them. Large HSAs would also give employers who cannot offer health insurance the opportunity to offer some tax-free health benefits.

Some budget analysts may be concerned about possible revenue losses from creating large HSAs. But every dollar lost to the Treasury would represent one or more dollars set aside in individual workers' HSAs. These funds would be set aside for workers' future health care expenses. With Medicare facing huge unfunded liabilities, large and growing HSAs would help make up the future funding gap in elderly health care. Moreover, capping the now-unlimited tax break for employer-sponsored coverage could increase federal revenues over time.

Large HSAs would help control health care costs, infuse competition into the medical marketplace, and give Americans ownership of their health care dollars.

A New Option: A Standard Deduction for Health Insurance

In 2007, President George W. Bush proposed a novel way to reform the tax treatment of health insurance and to reduce government interference in private-sector health care. The president proposed replacing the current, unlimited exclusion for employer-sponsored insurance with a "standard deduction for health insurance." Starting in 2009, individuals who purchased health insurance would receive a "standard deduction" of $7,500. Families who did so would receive a deduction of $15,000. Like the current exclusion, the standard deduction for health insurance would be deductible against both income and payroll taxes.

Yet the standard deduction for health insurance would be unlike the current exclusion in three important ways. First, it would be available to everyone, regardless of where they purchase health insurance. It would therefore eliminate discrimination against those without employer-sponsored coverage. Second, the standard deduction would not be an unlimited tax break; it would essentially be capped at $7,500 for individuals and $15,000 for families. (Those amounts would be indexed for inflation.) Third, anyone who purchased just a basic, catastrophic health insurance policy would receive the *full* $7,500 or $15,000 deduction. In other words, consumers would receive an enormous tax break for purchasing a basic, catastrophic insurance policy. But beyond that, the tax code would offer no incentive to purchase additional coverage. Whereas the current exclusion provides a constant incentive to purchase more and more coverage, the standard deduction would eliminate that distortion at the margin.

In certain respects, the president's proposal resembles large HSAs. It would level the playing field between individually purchased coverage and employer-sponsored insurance. It would eliminate incentives to purchase excessive coverage. Finally, it would cap the currently unlimited exclusion for employer-sponsored health insurance, and ultimately facilitate tax neutrality for health care.

Some conservatives have expressed concern that a standard deduction for health insurance in effect would increase taxes on those whose health benefits cost more than the amount of the standard deductions. Though that's troubling, it is by no means certain. In fact, those workers might not face a net tax increase at all, because the president's proposal would reduce other costs on those same workers. One such "tax" is the higher health care costs that result from the current exclusion. The standard deduction would reduce that tax. Another is the penalty imposed on workers who do not buy coverage through an employer. The standard deduction proposal would eliminate that tax as well.

Finally, when premiums exceeded the proposed deductions, employers could reduce health benefits and shift the difference to other untaxed compensation, such as contributions to HSAs, life insurance, or 401(k)s. That would leave those workers with zero additional tax liability. Or employers could shift that difference to wages, in which case the workers would pay taxes on it, but their take-home pay would rise.

A standard deduction for health insurance would dramatically reduce government interference in the health care sector. To illustrate, consider that HSAs were enacted to reduce government interference in consumers' health care decisions. Yet in a world where the standard deduction replaced the exclusion, HSAs would *increase*—rather than reduce—such interference. Although President Bush proposed preserving HSAs, reformers could garner additional support for a standard deduction—as well as achieve a better policy outcome—by signaling their willingness to trade away HSAs.

Large HSAs and a standard deduction for health insurance each has relative strengths. For example, large HSAs would give workers immediate control over the dollars that purchase their health benefits. With a standard deduction, workers could get temporarily short-changed if they purchase coverage on their own or if their employer drops coverage. Large HSAs would offer tax relief to the uninsurable, while a standard deduction would effectively penalize those who do not or cannot purchase insurance. However, a standard deduction would eliminate any tax-based price distortions at the margin, while large HSAs would preserve a price distortion at the margin. Nevertheless, each would facilitate further tax reforms that would eliminate government interference in consumers' health care decisions. Large HSAs and a standard deduction for health insurance thereby give reformers two promising options for reforming health care.

6. Government Health Programs

Government subsidizes medical care for some 100 million Americans through Medicare, Medicaid, and other programs. Rather than subsidize beneficiaries directly, government typically subsidizes them indirectly by delivering subsidies to health care providers when the beneficiary receives care. Government health programs exhibit all the negative effects of overreliance on health coverage, including moral hazard, reduced sensitivity to price and quality, and less competition. In addition, government sets payment rates for providers who treat beneficiaries in these programs. These gov-ernment price controls create additional waste and obstacles to competition and innovation. As the Federal Trade Commission (FTC) and Department of Justice (DOJ) recommend, government health care subsidies should be delivered directly to the intended beneficiaries. Allowing these patients to control their own health care dollars would secure them higher-quality care, minimize the harmful effects of excessive coverage, and obviate the need for government price controls.

Price Controls

Market prices convey information to producers and consumers about the cost of providing billions of items, how highly the items are valued by others, and how the available supply compares with existing need. Even with the most sophisticated tools conceivable, bureaucracies cannot replicate market prices because they cannot capture the information that producers and consumers reveal when they buy and sell items at unregulated prices. Even if a bureaucracy could capture all the necessary information for a point in time, conditions like supply, technology, and consumer preferences change too rapidly to update that information accurately.

When setting prices for services under government health programs, governments err in one of two ways: setting prices too high or too low. Setting prices too high results in resources being wasted

81

on services that provide less value than their cost. Setting prices too low results in shortages. As the FTC explains, "Paying too much wastes resources, while paying too little reduces both output and capacity, lowers the quality of the services that are provided, and diminishes the incentives for innovation."[1] Though intended to be a cost-containment tool,[2] price controls may actually increase costs.

Moreover, "Government-administered pricing . . . inadvertently can distort market competition."[3] According to the Commission, "One unintended consequence of [Medicare's] administered pricing systems has been to make some hospital services extraordinarily lucrative and others unprofitable. As a result, some services are more available (and others less available) than they would be in a competitive market."[4] As Columbia University law professor William Sage notes, "Public purchasing distorts prices, overbuilds capacity, and skews the development and dissemination of technology."[5]

For example, until 2003, Medicare payments to ambulatory surgery centers (ASCs) were based on a 1986 survey of ASC costs. Despite advances that increased productivity and reduced costs at such centers, Medicare's payments were not readjusted for 16 years (other than for inflation).[6] As a result, Medicare's overpayments encouraged growth and utilization of ASCs beyond the value they provided. Productivity gains in the provision of cardiovascular care quickly rendered Medicare payment rates excessive and encouraged overreliance on these services as well. "This pricing distortion creates a direct economic incentive for specialized cardiac hospitals to enter the market; such entry reflects areas that government pricing makes most profitable, which may or may not reflect consumers' needs and preferences."[7] Thus, taxpayers were billed more for these services than a competitive market would charge.

Government price controls also drive pricing for private payors. As former Medicare administrator Tom Scully has remarked,

> Medicare and Medicaid are such dominant players that the private sector has been forced to follow along—shadow pricing [Medicare's price controls] in recent years . . . In the long run, government price fixing for services has never worked in any system in any society, and I don't think it can work here, either. Having federal price fixing, no consumer information or pricing sensitivity, and no measurement of quality has led to predictable results: artificially high prices and uneven quality.[8]

Specialty Hospitals

Such price distortions also lead to further government obstacles to competition. Many large hospitals use excessive payments from public purchasers—notably Medicare—to subsidize other costs. These other costs can include legal requirements to provide care to those who cannot or will not pay, underpayments for other services, or the hospitals' own inefficiencies.

As a result, other providers, such as smaller specialty hospitals, have emerged to capture those excessive payments. These smaller hospitals compete by performing a smaller number of lucrative services at greater volume. Since specialty hospitals do not need to subsidize other costs, they can apply overpayments to higher staff compensation and superior service that pulls patients away from larger hospitals.[9]

In response, large hospitals have responded by lobbying for regulatory barriers to protect their position. In 2003, larger hospitals persuaded Congress to impose a temporary moratorium on the construction of new specialty hospitals even though a later study found that most large hospitals remain profitable in spite of competition.[10]

As the FTC and DOJ observe, "Competition . . . does not work well when certain facilities are expected to use higher profits in certain areas to cross-subsidize uncompensated care."[11] Specialty hospitals are an example of competition attempting to break through a highly regulated market. Competitors whose position is threatened respond with the coin of the realm.

Subsidies that go directly to the beneficiary would avoid the problems of excessive coverage, price controls, and much rent-seeking. In their report on competition in the health care system, the FTC and DOJ emphasized the importance of subsidizing individuals directly and making those subsidies transparent, rather than subsidizing institutions or providing hidden subsidies:

> The existence of subsidies and cross-subsidies complicates any plan to give consumers better price information and increase their price sensitivity. . . . Governments should reexamine the role of subsidies in health care markets in light of their inefficiencies and potential to distort competition. . . . In general, it is more efficient to provide subsidies directly to those who should receive them, rather than to obscure cross subsidies and indirect subsidies in transactions that are not transparent.[12]

Reforming government health programs to make subsidies transparent and direct to the intended beneficiaries would allow medical prices to be set by markets, reduce wasteful health spending and other distortions, and lead to lower-cost, higher-quality care for patients inside and outside of such programs.

Medicare

Medicare is the compulsory federal health program for elderly and disabled Americans, enacted in 1965 as part of former president Lyndon B. Johnson's "Great Society" agenda. Some 42 million Americans receive subsidized medical care through the program. The price of these subsidies is escalating to the point that existing resources will not be able to finance promised benefits to seniors.

Medicare subsidizes both hospital and physician care for Americans who reach age 65. It is financed through beneficiary premiums, dedicated taxes, transfers from state governments, and general federal revenues. Beneficiary premiums account for roughly 10 percent of overall costs.[13] A 2.9 percent payroll tax and a portion of the income taxes paid on Social Security benefits finance the hospital insurance portion of Medicare.

Medicare is compulsory for seniors as well as taxpayers. Seniors who opt out of Medicare's hospital insurance program are forced to forfeit all Social Security benefits, past and future.[14] Moreover, Medicare exhibits many of the worst effects of third-party control. Benefits are determined not by individual choice but through the political process. Despite language in the first section of the original Medicare law that states "nothing [in the Medicare law] shall be construed to authorize any federal officer or employee to exercise any supervision or control over . . . the selection . . . or compensation of any . . . person providing health services,"[15] Medicare routinely restricts seniors' choice of providers and sets prices for health services. Every year, Medicare beneficiaries waste billions of taxpayer dollars on poor-quality medical care. As a result, the costs of the Medicare program are growing rapidly and unsustainably.

Medicare and Freedom of Choice

Medicare is often referred to as a voluntary program. In fact, Medicare greatly restricts the freedom of workers, seniors, and the medical community. Even if Medicare neither crowded out other health insurance options for seniors, nor forced seniors who decline

Medicare benefits to forfeit all past and future Social Security benefits, funding Medicare would still be compulsory for all Americans forced to pay federal taxes that finance the program.

Medicare restricts Americans' freedom to purchase health insurance and medical care in countless ways. When it was enacted, Medicare essentially destroyed a large and growing market for retiree health insurance. According to Institute for Health Freedom president Sue Blevins, "In the 10 years before Medicare's enactment, the number of retirees with health insurance nearly doubled," reaching 60 percent by 1962.[16]

Medicare benefits are not a matter of individual choice, but are instead dictated to seniors through the political process. Whether an item is covered by Medicare often depends solely on who runs the Medicare bureaucracy.[17] One result of this process is that Medicare benefits lag behind private sector innovations. Medicare benefits were modeled on BlueCross/BlueShield coverage in 1965. In the 1970s, the Blues and other private insurers responded to consumer demand by adopting outpatient prescription drug coverage. Yet such coverage could only be added to Medicare by an act of Congress, as it was in 2003. Many seniors have purchased drug coverage through private, "Medicare supplemental" insurance; yet even the content of these plans is heavily regulated by Congress. Seniors have few options other than fee-for-service Medicare, and those options must provide the standard Medicare benefits package and are often canceled when Medicare payments to the private plans fall. Seniors who purchase coverage to supplement their Medicare benefits are restricted to 10 plans whose benefits are defined by law.

Medicare also restricts the right of beneficiaries to choose their own doctor. Medicare beneficiaries are effectively prohibited from going outside the Medicare program to purchase covered services from their own physicians. Doctors who participate in such arrangements are barred from the Medicare program for two years, which presents sufficient hardship to them to preclude the option for their patients. Americans with private health insurance and even Britons covered by the United Kingdom's socialized National Health Service may make such private arrangements with their doctors. Yet Medicare beneficiaries who seek treatment from their doctor outside of Medicare, perhaps because they prefer not to have a particular claim on file with the government, are effectively forbidden from exercising the same right.

Does Medicare Encourage Waste?

Because Medicare insulates beneficiaries from the costs of their health care decisions, it encourages patients to consume medical care even if such care provides little or no value. Elliot Fisher of Dartmouth Medical School examined regional variations in Medicare spending by beneficiaries with hip fractures, colorectal cancer, and heart attacks. According to Fisher and his co-authors,

> Residents of high-spending regions received 60% more care but did not have lower mortality rates, better functional status, or higher satisfaction . . . these differences in spending were explained almost entirely by greater frequency of physician visits, more frequent use of specialist consultations, more frequent tests and minor procedures, and greater use of the hospital and intensive care unit in high-spending regions.[18]

From their study of regional variations in Medicare spending, Fisher and his Dartmouth colleagues Jonathan Skinner and John Wennberg estimated that "nearly 20 percent of total Medicare expenditures . . . appears to provide no benefit in terms of survival, nor is it likely that this extra spending improves the quality of life."[19] That suggests that in 2007, Medicare will spend roughly $86 billion on unnecessary health services that do nothing to improve health.[20] It is important to note that this figure only includes services that provide no demonstrable benefit. It does not include additional sums spent on care that provides less benefit than its cost, that is, services that seniors would decline if they had the option of spending the money elsewhere. Therefore, $86 billion is a conservative estimate of the amount of Medicare spending that is wasted each year.

Does Medicare Deliver High-Quality Care?

One reason why so much Medicare spending accomplishes so little is that Medicare beneficiaries often do not receive the best available care. One study estimated that for 16 indicators, seniors received recommended care less than two-thirds of the time.[21] Drug manufacturers argue that underuse of antihypertensive drugs among Medicare patients leads to tens of thousands of premature deaths.[22]

Some studies have even found a *negative* correlation between higher Medicare spending and health care quality. Dartmouth economist Katherine Baicker and physician Amitabh Chandra found that additional spending "is not merely uncorrelated with the quality of care provided" but "negatively correlated with the use of effective care."[23] "Where does the money in high-spending states go, if not to highly effective care?" they ask. "It seems to be spent on expensive health care that has not been shown to have a positive effect on patient satisfaction or health outcomes."[24]

Medicare's poor performance in this area stems from a payment system that provides no incentive for providers to compete on the basis of quality. Tom Scully notes that within a region, Medicare pays "the exact same amount for hip replacement and the same amount for a heart bypass, if you're the best hospital or the worst hospital."[25] The FTC and DOJ observe that Medicare "do[es] not reward providers who deliver higher quality care or punish providers who deliver lower quality care."[26] MedPAC reports that Medicare's payment system "is largely neutral or negative towards quality . . . At times providers are paid even more when quality is worse, such as when complications occur as the result of error. In the [Medicare Advantage] program, some types of plans are held to higher standards than others, but paid the same, potentially creating disincentives for investing in quality."[27]

The Tax Burden of Medicare

The dynamic of excessive coverage via government subsidies has caused Medicare spending to grow rapidly since its inception. Despite official projections in 1965 that hospital insurance under Medicare would cost only $9 billion in 1990, actual spending in 1990 was $66 billion.[28] Medicare payroll taxes are now nearly double what its sponsors promised would be necessary, having been raised at least eight times since its creation and most recently in 1994.[29] In addition, the program consumes a growing share of general revenue.

Medicare spending is expected to increase even more dramatically in the future, fueled by the retirement of the baby-boom generation, rising longevity, rising medical prices, and new medical technologies. In 2007, the Board of Trustees that oversees the Medicare program made several predictions about future Medicare growth:[30]

- "Total Medicare expenditures were $408 billion in 2006 and are expected to increase in future years at a faster pace than either workers' earnings or the economy overall.
- "As a percentage of GDP, expenditures are projected to increase from 3.1 percent currently to 11.3 percent by 2080. . . .
- "The level of Medicare expenditures is expected to exceed that for Social Security in 2028 and, by 2081, to be 80 percent more than the cost of Social Security.
- "Growth of this magnitude, if realized, would place a substantially greater strain on the nation's workers, Medicare beneficiaries, and the Federal Budget."

Exacerbating these cost pressures will be the fact that the number of workers paying taxes to support Medicare is declining relative to the number of seniors and disabled drawing subsidies. Today, there are roughly four workers paying into the Medicare program for every beneficiary. According to Medicare's trustees, there will be only 2.4 workers per beneficiary in 2030 and two workers per beneficiary by 2079 (see Figure 6.1).[31]

Figure 6.1
MEDICARE WORKER-TO-BENEFICIARY RATIO

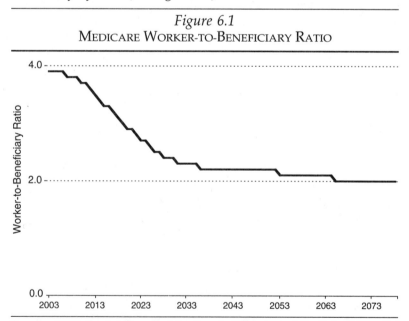

SOURCE: *2005 Annual Report of the Board of Trustees of the Federal Hospital Insurance and Federal Supplementary Medical Insurance Trust Funds* (Washington: Government Printing Office, March 23, 2005), p. 57.

Figure 6.2
MEDICARE'S UNFUNDED LIABILITIES COMPARED
WITH OTHER MEASURES, 2007
(IN TRILLIONS)

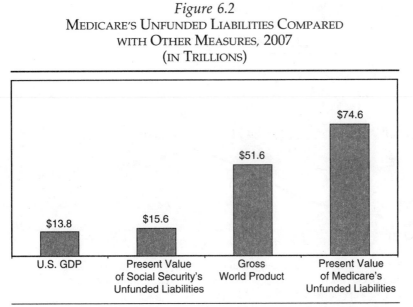

SOURCES: International Monetary Fund, World Economic Outlook Database, April 2007; *2007 Annual Report of the Board of Trustees of the Federal Old-Age and Survivors Insurance and Disability Insurance Trust Funds* (Washington: Government Printing Office, April 23, 2007), p. 61; and *2007 Annual Report of the Board of Trustees of the Federal Hospital Insurance and Federal Supplementary Medical Insurance Trust Funds* (Washington: Government Printing Office, May 1, 2007), pp. 67, 105, 120.

As noted earlier, the federal government would have to deposit approximately $74.6 trillion in an interest-bearing account to cover all of Medicare's future unfunded liabilities. That sum is larger than the combined GDPs of all the nations on earth ($51.6 trillion in 2004),[32] five times greater than U.S. GDP,[33] and nearly five times the amount required to cover Social Security's future deficits (see Figure 6.2).[34]

A large portion of this burden is the prescription drug benefit added to Medicare by President Bush and Congress in 2003. The drug benefit alone accounts for nearly one-fourth of Medicare's future fiscal imbalance.[35] According to former Medicare trustee Tom Saving, the prescription drug benefit "represents the largest expansion of elderly entitlements since the passage of Medicare almost 40 years ago."[36] New York University law professor Daniel Shaviro

Figure 6.3
GENERAL REVENUE TRANSFERS TO MEDICARE AS A SHARE OF FEDERAL INCOME TAX REVENUE

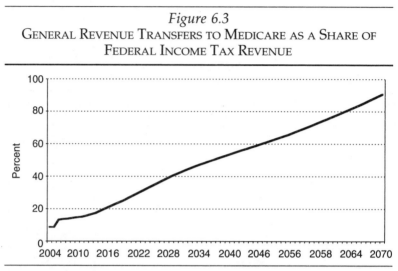

SOURCE: Andrew J. Rettenmaier and Thomas R. Saving, "The 2004 Medicare and Social Security Trustees Reports," National Center for Policy Analysis Policy Report no. 266, June 2004, p. 6.

calls the Medicare prescription drug benefit "a straight tax increase on future generations."[37] Economics columnist Robert Samuelson calls the measure "one of the worst pieces of social legislation in decades."[38] According to U.S. Comptroller General David Walker, "The prescription drug bill was probably the most fiscally irresponsible piece of legislation since the 1960s."[39]

The Impact of Medicare's Growing Tax Burden

Current law promises Medicare beneficiaries far more than current revenue streams can provide. In 2004, Medicare required a transfer from general federal revenues equal to almost 9 percent of federal income tax revenue.[40] Absent any changes to Medicare benefits or financing, Medicare will require general revenue transfers equal to 25 percent of income tax revenue by 2030, and 50 percent of income tax revenue by 2040 (see Figure 6.3).[41]

In 2004, Cato Institute senior fellow Jagadeesh Gokhale estimated that covering Medicare's future deficits through higher taxes would require increasing the Medicare payroll tax in 2004 from 2.9 percent to 17.8 percent of all wages—more than a 500 percent increase. If Congress fails to make any changes to Medicare until 2008, the required payroll tax rate would be 19.8 percent—nearly a 700 percent increase.[42]

The burden of the taxes required to cover Medicare's deficits would be even higher than these estimates suggest. According to Harvard economist Martin Feldstein, "The problem of the increasing cost of Medicare is not just the extra real resources that will be devoted to improving the health of the aged but also the deadweight loss of the higher taxes that would be needed to finance that spending if we continue to rely on the pay-as-you-go tax system."[43] Feldstein estimates that the forgone economic benefits would be equal to about two-thirds of the amount raised, "making the total burden of the extra spending nearly twice as large as the additional health resource costs."[44] In other words, an increase in the Medicare payroll tax of 14.9 percentage points (from 2.9 percent to 17.8 percent) would carry a total cost equal to nearly 25 percent of wages.

Staying the present course would impose enormous burdens on current and future taxpayers. This makes reforming Medicare not just necessary, but urgent.

Reforming Medicare

America's seniors have a right to choose their health insurance, their doctors, and the medical treatments their health care dollars can purchase. America's workers have the right to control their own savings and plan for their own health needs in retirement. They do not deserve to have an ever-growing share of their earnings confiscated to support a Medicare program that breeds waste and restricts their freedom. Protecting taxpayers and improving the quality of health care for seniors requires fundamental reform of the Medicare program. Congress should allow seniors to opt out of Medicare entirely without loss of Social Security benefits, as well as on a case-by-case basis through private contracts with their doctors. In addition, Medicare should be overhauled to subsidize seniors directly, to give them true choice among competing private health plans, and to allow today's workers to prefund Medicare's obligations through personal accounts.

Rather than have their health care dollars meted out to them, seniors should have the opportunity to take their health care dollars into the marketplace to purchase coverage of their choice. Congress should move Medicare from its current system of defined benefits to a system of defined contributions. Under this model, Medicare would subsidize each beneficiary directly in the form of a voucher that beneficiaries would use to purchase health coverage from among competing private plans. Seniors could add their own funds to the voucher to purchase a health plan of their choice. To minimize bias toward excessive coverage, beneficiaries could use part of the voucher to purchase health insurance and deposit the rest into a health savings account.

Ownership of their benefits would make seniors more price-sensitive and encourage them to eliminate the sizable amounts of waste in the program, because doing so would be in each beneficiary's financial interest. As noted earlier, studies have documented wide geographical variations in per beneficiary Medicare spending. Elliott Fisher reports that Medicare spends more than $10,000 per beneficiary in Manhattan, but less than $5,000 per beneficiary in Portland, Oregon.[45] Moreover, higher Medicare spending is often correlated with lower-quality care. If Medicare vouchers were based on consumption patterns in lower-cost/higher-quality regions (and adjusted for regional cost-of-living differences), they would encourage seniors in high-spending regions to eliminate unnecessary expenditures and would force providers in high-spending regions to emulate their more efficient colleagues. Subsidizing seniors directly also would encourage insurers to focus exclusively on the needs of their customers, leading to greater competition and innovation among insurers.

While seniors with higher medical costs likely would be charged higher premiums, Congress could take steps to guarantee that all seniors would be able to obtain coverage. First, Congress could adjust vouchers according to risk. Seniors in worse health could receive larger subsidies to ensure they would be able to afford health insurance.

Second, Congress could further reduce incentives for insurers to avoid seriously ill seniors by encouraging long-term insurance contracts instead of the one-year contracts currently offered by private Medicare plans. Tom Saving and Andrew Rettenmaier point out that all seniors tend to consume similar amounts of medical care in their last year of life. Yet those who are less healthy at age 65 tend not to live as long as healthier seniors. Those who are healthiest at age 65 will live several years before they begin to incur end-of-life medical costs, and will incur low-to-moderate medical expenses in those intervening years. As a result, the beneficiaries who cost Medicare the most over the long term are those who are healthiest when they enroll at age 65. Therefore, longer-term insurance contracts would put healthy and less-than-healthy beneficiaries on a more equal footing when choosing private Medicare plans.

Additional measures could further protect seniors who incur high medical bills from being neglected by private insurers. Seniors who enroll in a long-term Medicare contract could remain with the insurer as long as they wish. To prevent insurers from underserving the sickest patients, Congress could allow beneficiaries to switch to another private insurance plan whenever they choose. If the new plan would not accept the beneficiary's voucher as payment in full, the old plan could be required to make a severance payment to the new plan; the amount of this payment would be set by the new plan. Because the beneficiary's decision to switch health plans would require the former insurer to pay a competitor whatever that competitor demands, private insurers would be heavily discouraged from underserving sicker patients. Moreover, this would preserve the beneficiaries' freedom of choice, and lead to greater competition among insurers on the basis of price and quality.[46] Used in tandem, risk-adjusted vouchers and long-term contracts would give the federal government complementary tools to protect seniors from adverse screening decisions by insurers.

It is unlikely that Congress would allow Medicare's growth to crowd out other areas of government spending, such as national defense. It is equally unlikely that Congress, even over many years, would be able to increase taxes as dramatically as will become necessary to maintain existing benefit levels. Thus it is almost certain that Congress will have to cut Medicare benefits. Giving seniors control over their Medicare benefits would allow them to retain the benefits that mean the most to them, rather than have those benefits taken away through the political process.

Prefunding Medicare?

Even with direct subsidies, greater choice, and competition, Medicare would still rest on the shaky foundation of intergenerational financing by which taxes on the young pay the medical bills of the old. Moreover, the program still would not give beneficiaries full ownership over their health care dollars.

As nations around the world are learning, pay-as-you-go financing schemes are increasingly burdensome for successive generations. First, they are subject to generational shocks. As noted earlier, when the U.S. baby-boom generation retires, the number of workers supporting each Medicare beneficiary will drop from 4 to 2.4 by 2030. Baby boomers are currently paying for their parents' Medicare coverage, but this tax burden is light compared with the one baby boomers will impose on their children and grandchildren. Second, there is a tendency for each generation of seniors to demand additional benefits for which they have not paid. The new Medicare prescription drug subsidies are a case in point.

As the per-beneficiary cost of Medicare grows, this pyramid scheme will become as unsustainable as any other. Eugene Steuerle and Adam Carasso of the Urban Institute estimate that under current law *all* retirees will receive far more in Medicare benefits than they paid into the program during their working years. A one-earner couple that retired in 2005 on a salary of $70,000 will receive $222,000 more than they contributed. Such net transfers are higher for lower-income retirees, yet even high-income retirees walk away with more than they put in. A dual-earner couple retiring on a salary of $280,000 will receive a net transfer of nearly $100,000. The amount of these transfers will grow over time, approaching $1 million for many future low-income retirees.[47]

Medicare's pay-as-you-go financing structure also discourages saving and reduces economic growth. As Rettenmaier and Saving observe, "The current generation-transfer system of financing Medicare ... results in a reduction in the nation's capital stock and in national income."[48]

Moreover, the above-mentioned reforms would still leave control over seniors' retirement health benefits in the hands of politicians. Even if Medicare beneficiaries may choose from competing private plans and HSAs encourage them to be more prudent consumers, the vouchers that enable them to purchase private coverage or fund their HSAs would be subject to the political process. The amount of these vouchers could be reduced by Congress at any time. With the enormous unfunded liabilities facing Medicare, and the likelihood that workers will resist the tax increases required to maintain current benefits, it is inevitable that Congress will someday have to reduce Medicare benefits. Vouchers can help seniors preserve the health coverage that means the most to them. However, vouchers do not provide the protection of real ownership. Though greater choice and competition can help, seniors' health benefits will not be fully secured until seniors own the dollars that purchase those benefits—not just in the form of a check from the government, but from the moment those dollars are earned.

In response to these shortcomings, prominent economists have recommended giving workers ownership over their Medicare benefits from day one. Individuals would deposit some or all of their Medicare payroll taxes into personal savings accounts dedicated exclusively to their medical expenses in retirement. Over time, those funds would grow and be able to provide their owners with the benefits that Medicare's current financing scheme cannot. Workers who do not earn enough to provide for a minimum level of health coverage would receive subsidies into their accounts from the federal government. In essence, individual savings accounts and the power of compound interest would prefund Medicare's future obligations.

Before Congress and President Bush created Medicare's prescription drug benefit, Harvard's Martin Feldstein estimated that annual Medicare personal account deposits "equal to about 1.4% of total payroll would eventually be enough to pay for the full increase in the cost of Medicare, obviating a nine percentage point payroll tax increase." He writes, "in the long run [retiree health accounts] would eliminate the need for massive taxes that would otherwise reduce disposable income of low- and middle-income workers by 20 percent and impose an extra deadweight loss equal to more than six percent of existing wages."[49]

Prefunding Medicare through personal savings accounts would minimize the cost of meeting existing Medicare obligations. By 2007, Medicare had incurred $75 trillion in unfunded liabilities to future retirees. These obligations are implicit debt in that they do not appear in the federal budget. Rettenmaier and Saving estimate that prefunding what are now only implicit obligations would fulfill those obligations at a lower cost. "[I]f we embark on a transition to a prepaid system," they write, "the total resource commitment will be reduced."[50] Before the enactment of the new Medicare prescription drug benefit, they estimated that the annual cost of a prefunded system would exceed the costs of the current pay-as-you-go system for 16 years. After that point, the pay-as-you-go system becomes and remains more costly.[51] They note that the costs are greater the longer Congress waits, and that Congress should move to a pre-funded system while baby boomers are still in the labor force and in their peak earning years.

In the short term, depositing workers' payroll taxes into their own personal accounts would reduce federal tax revenues. Congress would have three options for managing the revenue loss: increase taxes, borrow, or reduce spending. Some have suggested raising taxes to restore this revenue,[52] yet the additional deadweight losses make this response unwise. Restoring the lost revenue with bor-rowed funds is tantamount to a future tax increase, and would defeat the purpose of prefunding Medicare obligations by leaving the implicit debt of the federal government unchanged. The best option is for Congress to reduce spending elsewhere.

Medicaid

Medicaid is the largest means-tested public program in the nation. Enacted in 1965, it provides medical care to millions of low-income Americans. It also does much more. Medicaid encourages the poor—and the not-so-poor—to become dependent on government. It encourages them to behave in ways that increase the cost of govern-ment and of health care, which makes self-reliance more difficult for their neighbors. And it encourages states to get more people to behave that way. Medicaid is a program in desperate need of reform. More than reform, however, Medicaid needs to be cut down to size.

How Medicaid Operates

Medicaid subsidizes health care for low-income Americans. The federal government and state and territorial governments jointly administer Medicaid—or more precisely, 56 separate Medicaid pro-grams.[53] Participation is ostensibly voluntary for states. No state is required to participate, though all states do. Each state's Medicaid program must provide a federally defined set of health benefits to a federally defined population of eligible individuals. States can expand eligibility and benefits beyond the minimum federal require-ments. In 1997, the federal government created the State Children's Health Insurance Program (SCHIP), which allowed states to expand their Medicaid programs to include (or to enact a parallel and more flexible program for) children in families with incomes slightly higher than the cutoff for Medicaid eligibility.

In return, each state receives federal funds in proportion to what it spends. The more a state spends on its Medicaid program, the more it receives from the federal government. The ratio of federal-to-state contributions, or "match," is determined according to a state's relative wealth: poorer states receive a higher match, wealthier states receive a lower match. On average, 57 percent of Medicaid funding comes from the federal government and 43 percent comes from the states.

For beneficiaries, Medicaid is an entitlement. So long as individuals meet the eligibility criteria, they have a legally enforceable right to benefits. Medicaid typically offers services to beneficiaries free of charge.[54] It primarily serves four low-income groups: mothers and their children, the disabled, the elderly, and those needing long-term care. In 2004, Medicaid served a total of about 60 million Americans, including some 44 million low-income children and their parents and 16 million elderly and disabled beneficiaries.[55] Although the vast majority of Medicaid *beneficiaries* are low-income children and their families, the vast majority of Medicaid *spending* goes to the elderly and disabled, who use far more care than their younger counterparts. In 2003, Medicaid spent $1,410 per covered child, compared with an average of $11,659 per disabled beneficiary and $10,147 per elderly beneficiary. The elderly and disabled account for 70 percent of Medicaid spending. Medicaid provides supplemental subsidies for approximately six million Medicare beneficiaries who account for 40 percent of Medicaid spending, and Medicaid finances nearly half of all nursing home care in the United States.[56] In addition to benefits provided to those enrolled in the program, Medicaid's Disproportionate Share Hospital program provides added federal funding to hospitals that treat a disproportionate share of uninsured patients.

Doctors' participation in Medicaid is voluntary. Like Medicare, Medicaid pays for physician care and other covered expenses according to fixed prices that are set administratively by government bureaucracies. Medicaid payments to providers are typically lower than those under Medicare, and are well below payments from private payers.

The Tax Burden of Medicaid

Medicaid imposes a growing burden on taxpayers due to a number of factors that are driving growth in Medicaid spending. A large

Figure 6.4
TOTAL MEDICAID SPENDING, 1970–2005

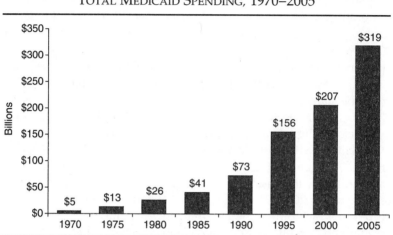

SOURCE: National Association of State Budget Officers, "2005 State Expenditure Report," Fall 2006, p. 47.

share comes from persistent expansions of state Medicaid programs. Encouraged by federal SCHIP funds and overflowing tax coffers, states expanded their Medicaid programs in the 1990s.[57] Another source of spending growth is the rising cost of medical care. Related to this, many argue that the rising cost of private health insurance and the resulting growth in the number of Americans without private health insurance lead to greater Medicaid enrollment and spending. Finally, as the population ages and longevity increases, more Americans are relying on Medicaid to provide nursing home and other long-term care.

Medicaid spending continues to grow faster than all other state budget items and now accounts for almost 23 percent of state spending.[58] The National Association of State Budget Officers has projected that in 2006, total Medicaid spending continued to surpass elementary and secondary education as the largest item in state budgets (see Figure 6.4).[59] The National Association of State Budget Officers reports, "Even after a full economic recovery is under way for state budgets, increases in Medicaid costs will far outstrip the growth in state revenues into the future."[60]

Does Medicaid Encourage Waste?

Medicaid's most obvious effect is the access to medical care it provides its beneficiaries. Evaluating the Medicaid bargain, however, requires a tally of all its effects, seen and unseen.[61]

Medicaid encourages overutilization of medical care by recipients. The program typically offers services to beneficiaries free of charge, which encourages beneficiaries to consume medical care without regard to its cost. Lee Anne Fennell of the University of Illinois observes that a recipient in this position "would be expected to consume medical services right up to the point at which she obtains no benefit from them." Fennell describes this as overutilization because it diverts money away from more productive uses, such as medical care that would have benefited someone else more. Fennell explains, "Although at first blush one might think this is the appropriate amount of health care to consume, where resources are limited each marginal dollar spent on health care . . . should be spent on the individual who can gain the most from it. When money no longer serves as a mode of expressing how much a particular service is valued, there is no way to know whether providing that service to a given individual represents the most efficient use of limited resources."[62]

Though Medicaid encourages some 50 million Americans to overutilize medical care, data on the extent of overutilization and its costs are scarce. If overutilization in Medicaid is consistent with research regarding overutilization in Medicare, overutilization in Medicaid also could exceed $50 billion per year.[63]

This affects, and is affected by, other costs of the program. One way overutilization can affect the magnitude of other costs is by increasing the prices of medical goods and services. Encouraging 50 million Americans to consume care with little regard to cost should result in an increase in demand for medical services. This in turn should result in an increase in price, making medical care more costly for both public and private payers.

Medicaid's Unseen Costs: Price Controls

Medicaid's administered prices act as price controls, which typically pay doctors at below-market rates. Medicare's physician reimbursement rates are widely considered to be below market-clearing levels. Yet Medicaid pays doctors even less. By 1998, a doctor who treated a Medicaid patient was receiving just 62 percent of what that doctor would receive for treating a Medicare patient.[64]

As with all price ceilings, Medicaid's impose costs and lead to unintended consequences. One such unintended consequence is that doctors try to get around the price controls. Doctors whose patient base is at least 25 percent Medicaid patients are much more likely to manipulate reimbursement rules.[65] This can be done to obtain coverage for an otherwise noncovered service, or to increase the amount a physician is paid by generating additional claims.

Another cost of Medicaid's price controls is imposed on private purchasers of medical care. Mark Duggan of the University of Maryland and Fiona Scott Morton of Yale University estimate Medicaid increases the prices of non-Medicaid prescriptions by 13.3 percent over and above what they otherwise would be.[66] Thus, if a regime of medications costs a private payer $1,000 per year, more than $115 of that cost is attributable to Medicaid.

This constitutes a large yet unseen cost of the Medicaid program. Like overutilization, it influences other costs imposed by Medicaid. Increasing the price of medical goods and services for private payers necessarily increases the cost of private health insurance, particularly for those who are already Medicaid-eligible or are on the cusp of eligibility.

Medicaid's Unseen Costs: Discouraging Work and Savings

Another category of costs imposed by Medicaid come as a result of how individuals and institutions respond to the perverse incentives the program creates. For example, because Medicaid is a means-tested program, individuals lose eligibility if their income exceeds a certain amount. As a result, beneficiaries often avoid work and savings if it would mean losing Medicaid benefits. Likewise, potential beneficiaries often reduce work effort and savings in order to become eligible. These incentives pull many Americans toward poverty. Meanwhile, the tax burden imposed by Medicaid—which includes its effects on the cost of private medical care and insurance—makes the climb out of poverty more difficult for those who try.

Medicaid provides a typical beneficiary thousands of dollars of medical care each year. The prospect of losing Medicaid benefits can be a significant deterrent for individuals to enter the workforce or increase their incomes. University of Kentucky economist Aaron Yelowitz explains the effect Medicaid has on work incentives:

> Until 1987 the income eligibility limit (the maximum income allowable to receive benefits) for Aid to Families with Dependent Children was effectively the same as the income limit for Medicaid. This meant that at a predefined level of earnings, both AFDC and Medicaid benefits were lost. Losing Medicaid abruptly created a large and negative "notch" in income realized from work, totaling several thousand dollars. Because of this notch problem, a welfare recipient who increased her earnings above the income limit would actually make her family worse off than before. The notch contributed to keeping families dependent on welfare and discouraged the movement of welfare recipients into the workforce.[67]

Yelowitz observed, "Earnings need[ed] to more than double from the $9,000 level before total income approache[d] what it was before losing Medicaid."

Yelowitz confirmed that this disincentive to work affected the behavior of Medicaid recipients. He found that when income limits for Medicaid eligibility were raised in the late 1980s and early 1990s, enrollment in the Aid for Families with Dependent Children program fell. He posits this response came from skilled AFDC recipients who would no longer lose their Medicaid benefits if they returned to work. He estimates this was responsible for a 6.3 percent decline in AFDC caseloads.[68]

Since 1996, the link between AFDC (now Temporary Assistance for Needy Families) benefits and Medicaid benefits has been broken, as Medicaid income limits have been raised. Nonetheless, Medicaid still provides a disincentive to work; it has merely moved up the income scale with the eligibility cutoff. Yelowitz observes, "As states have expanded eligibility for Medicaid by increasing the income limit to a higher level . . . the notch has moved."[69]

Medicaid benefits can also be lost if one's assets exceed the allowable limits. Thus Medicaid also discourages individuals from accumulating savings. Yelowitz and MIT's Jonathan Gruber found that rather than save their earnings, nonelderly Medicaid beneficiaries increased consumption to remain eligible. They estimate that in 1993, Medicaid reduced asset holdings among those eligible by the equivalent of $1,600 to $2,000 per household in today's dollars.[70]

Substituting consumption for savings allows Medicaid beneficiaries to maintain their eligibility. However, it decreases the likelihood that they will escape poverty. These disincentives are likely to be even greater today, as a result of subsequent expansions of eligibility and benefits.

Medicaid's Unseen Costs: Crowd-Out

Just as Medicaid discourages self-help generally, it also discourages other efforts to provide medical care to recipients and potential recipients. This effect is typically referred to as "crowd-out." For instance, in most cases, the availability of matching federal funds should encourage states to increase medical assistance to the poor. However, states often use Medicaid revenue to displace effort they would otherwise exert themselves. Likewise, eligible individuals rely on Medicaid to finance their medical care rather than take steps to cover their own medical expenses. Medicaid crowds out private communal assistance, such as mutual aid, and purchasing of private health insurance. Medicaid also encourages nonrecipients to reduce charitable efforts to provide medical care to the needy. This may result because people believe that the problem of medical care for the poor is "taken care of" or because the burden of Medicaid makes taxpayers less able to donate to charity.

Anyone who meets federal eligibility criteria (regarding age, income, assets, etc.), or a particular state's broadened criteria, is entitled to Medicaid benefits. This encourages many to enroll even when they could obtain care and coverage elsewhere. Before the enactment of Medicaid, many working-class Americans financed their medical expenses with the help of fraternal organizations, also known as mutual-aid societies. According to historian David Beito, by 1920, such organizations "dominated the field of health insurance. They offered two basic varieties of protection: cash payments to compensate for income from working days lost and the care of a doctor. Some societies . . . founded tuberculosis sanitariums, specialist clinics, and hospitals." Beito writes, "A conservative estimate would be that one of three adult males was a member [of such organizations] in 1920, including a large segment of the working class." Moreover, these organizations "achieved a formidable presence among blacks and immigrant groups."[71]

Beito focuses on the effect that government medical assistance had on mutual-aid societies' efforts to provide medical care to low-income residents of the Mississippi Delta. "For twenty-five years before 1967," he writes, "thousands of low-income blacks in the Mississippi Delta obtained affordable hospital care through fraternal societies. Although there were clear deficiencies, the quality was reasonably good, especially given the limited resources. Most importantly, the Taborian Hospital and the Friendship Clinic excelled in providing benefits to patients that were not easily quantifiable, including personal attention, comfortable surroundings, and community pride. Both societies accomplished these feats with little outside help. The Knights and Daughters of Tabor and the United Order of Friendship of America forged extensive networks of mutual aid and self-help for thousands of low-income blacks."[72]

However, the advent of federal assistance changed the landscape. "In 1966 the federal Office of Economic Opportunity, the major front-line agency in the War on Poverty, entered the scene with subsidized health care." Beito writes, "The next year witnessed the end of fraternal hospitalization in the Delta." At the time, the leaders of the Knights and Daughters of Tabor wrote, "Since 90% of our membership is composed of people who are classified in the poverty category—they are eligible for free care at the Mound Bayou Community Hospital. Therefore, we are losing their membership in the order. This puts the Order in a declining position in membership and financial income." Beito continues, "The rapid inflow of federal money dampened the community's old habits of medical mutual aid and self-help. According to Dr. Louis Bernard of Meharry Medical College, 'The dollars available from the so-called antipoverty program ruined the International Order of the Knights and Daughters of Tabor.'"[73] Beito focused mainly on the effects of federal subsidies to create hospitals, not Medicaid explicitly. However, Medicaid accounts for a notable share of hospitals' income and was part of the changes that occurred during this period, having been enacted in 1965.[74] Medicaid could be presumed to have crowded out this type of private health insurance even if no other evidence of this tendency were available.

Yet, Medicaid also encourages employers of low-income workers not to offer coverage, and encourages low-income workers not to enroll in private coverage. Researchers at the Robert Wood Johnson

103

Foundation surveyed 22 leading studies on whether government coverage crowds out private coverage. The researchers concluded that crowd-out "seems inevitable." Although the scale of crowd-out varied, more than half of these studies found that expansions of public coverage were accompanied by reductions in private coverage. Some even found that enrollment growth in public programs was completely offset by reductions in private coverage.[75]

Medicaid discourages private insurance for nursing home and other long-term care expenses as well. Jeffrey Brown of the University of Illinois at Urbana-Champaign and Amy Finkelstein of the National Bureau of Economic Research found that 60 percent to 75 percent of the benefits from private long-term care insurance "are redundant of benefits that Medicaid would otherwise have paid." They estimate that Medicaid by itself discourages 66 percent to 90 percent of seniors from purchasing such insurance.[76]

Medicaid induces similar responses by states. In most cases, states can double their money by increasing their Medicaid contribution and obtaining additional federal funds. However, in certain cases, states are able to do better than doubling their money. Some states have used federal funds to supplant what they would have funded themselves.

The federal government's open-ended commitment to match state Medicaid spending alters a state's incentive to fund Medicaid relative to other priorities. States receive an average of $1.30 from Washington for every dollar they spend. Spending $1 on police buys $1 of police protection, but spending $1 on Medicaid buys $2.30 of health care. This encourages states to broaden their programs, even beyond what is necessary to assist the truly needy. According to the Urban Institute, 21 percent of eligible adults and 27 percent of eligible children have private coverage.[77] If nearly one-quarter of those who are eligible for Medicaid have private coverage despite their eligibility, this strongly suggests that states have expanded Medicaid beyond its original purpose of providing medical assistance to the truly needy.

In what some observers describe as "fiscal shenanigans," states have employed numerous accounting schemes to secure federal matching funds, which are then diverted from their Medicaid programs toward other priorities.[78] For example, the Disproportionate Share Hospital program was created to provide additional federal funding to hospitals that treat a large number of uninsured patients who cannot pay for their own care. Yet DSH funds often do not increase overall funding for uncompensated care. Instead, they often displace prior state spending. This effectively allows states to use federal Medicaid funds for expenditures having little or nothing to do with medical care for the poor. Duggan studied California's Medicaid DSH program and found that in 1990, "every dollar of DSH funds crowds out one dollar of [local] government subsidies."[79] Surveys have found that as much as one-third of federal DSH payments were captured by states and spent on other items.[80]

As one might expect, when such funds are diverted from the provision of care, they do little to improve health. According to Dartmouth economists Katherine Baicker and Douglas Staiger, "Surprisingly little is known about whether these public subsidies have had any impact on patient care, despite spending of nearly $200 billion during the 1990s on these programs by state and federal governments."[81] Duggan finds that "virtually none of the billions of dollars received by these facilities results in improved medical care quality for the poor."[82] He concludes, "health outcomes for low-income individuals did not improve despite a substantial increase in public medical spending for the indigent . . . If California's experience is representative of the United States as a whole, then the social benefit from this $20 billion increase in public medical spending has been much smaller than its cost."[83]

Such "fiscal shenanigans" are not so much an illness as a symptom. Common sense suggests that control over state programs should be left to local officials, who know more about the needs of their communities than distant federal officials. Although it is tempting to define such fiscal shenanigans as wasted spending, Medicaid funds diverted from medical care do not lose all value. In fact, Medicaid resources may do more good when they are diverted to other priorities than when spent in accordance with the dictates of federal legislators and bureaucrats. Baicker and Staiger note these funds "may result in other benefits to society . . . such as tax abatement or subsidies of other government programs."[84] However, the convoluted path those funds take results in unnecessary costs.

How Medicaid Affects Nonrecipients

Medicaid also imposes costs on nonbeneficiaries, including higher health care costs and a greater tax burden. Medicaid's per capita tax burden exceeds $1,000. This does not include hidden costs of the program, including higher prices for private purchasers. Even so, a tax burden of this magnitude poses a significant obstacle to those who would like to pull themselves out of poverty through self-help. On the one hand, this cost could discourage and frustrate self-help among recipients and potential recipients just as much as the availability of benefits does. On the other hand, the cost could be imposed mostly on higher-income earners. In this case, marginal tax rates for those in this group would be much higher, which would reduce work incentives for higher-income earners. How the tax burden of Medicaid is distributed will determine whether (and to what extent) the tax burden of Medicaid appears as a disincentive to work for the poor or for the non-poor.[85]

Does Medicaid Provide Quality Care?

The problems of crowd-out and Medicaid dependence become even graver when one considers the quality of care offered by Medicaid against that offered by private coverage.

Provider choice is one dimension of health coverage quality. One survey found the strongest predictor of dissatisfaction with a health plan, as measured by unwillingness to recommend the plan to others, is lack of choice with respect to providers.[86] Choice also influences the quality of care. If patients are unhappy with the care they are receiving from their physicians, the quality of their care will improve if they have other options. They are more likely to find a provider who meets their needs, and providers are more likely to compete with each other to do so.

Physicians unwilling to accept Medicaid's low reimbursement rates as payment in full must refuse Medicaid patients. As a result, many doctors do so. One study notes, "Physicians in states with the lowest Medicaid fees were less willing to accept most or all new Medicaid patients in both 1998 and 2003."[87] Beneficiaries often see their physician choices narrow even when payments to physicians rise. From 1998 to 2003, states increased physician payments by twice the rate of inflation.[88] Yet the share of doctors accepting all new Medicaid patients dropped from 48.1 percent to 39.4 percent from 1999 to 2003. The share of doctors accepting no new Medicaid patients increased from 26.4 percent to 30.5 percent over the same period.[89] This suggests that other features of the program restrict Medicaid patients' choice of doctors.

The costs of Medicaid's limited choices fall hardest on women. Medicaid subsidizes health care for 1 out of 10 American women, who comprise 71 percent of adult beneficiaries.[90] Women with Medicaid coverage have more difficulty finding a doctor than uninsured women and significantly more difficulty than women with private coverage. They are twice as likely as women with private coverage to have difficulty obtaining care due to a lack of doctors or clinics.[91]

How does Medicaid affect health outcomes? Medicaid certainly provides necessary and often emergent medical care to millions of recipients. However, a number of studies question whether the quality of care provided improves health outcomes as much as private alternatives.

A 1999 study by the National Bureau of Economic Research observed that "relatively little is known about the effects of Medicaid on health outcomes."[92] The authors note that "[f]indings from studies of Medicaid's effect on infant health are inconclusive," and that the only study to examine the program's effect on children's health found "implausibly large" reductions in child mortality and "either no effect or a negative effect on a mother's evaluation of her child's health (e.g., activity limitations)."[93] Although the authors set out to quantify the health benefits of Medicaid coverage, they found "at best weak support for the hypothesis that Medicaid improves the health of low-income children."[94] They concluded, "The proposition that health insurance is the cure for adverse health outcomes among poor and near-poor children has not been adequately demonstrated."[95] Regarding the federal government's creation of the State Children's Health Insurance Program, which "allocated $24.3 billion for the expansion of publicly provided health insurance, ostensibly to improve the health of low-income children," the authors commented, "It is remarkable that there is so little empirical evidence to support so large an expenditure."[96]

A study by researchers at Stanford University and the RAND Corporation found that HIV patients with health coverage are less likely to die prematurely, "but private insurance is more effective than public coverage. The better outcomes associated with private insurance are attributable to the more restrictive prescription drug policies of Medicaid."[97] The authors write:

> Some private insurers may place limits on when [they] will cover [highly active anti-retroviral therapy, or HAART], but

> Medicaid limits can be quite severe. Many states place limits on how many prescriptions can be filled per month, and since HAART therapy alone averages 4.8 prescriptions, these can limit coverage for not only HAART but also drugs to treat opportunistic infections associated with advanced disease. Many of the drugs also required prior authorization that restricted use to advanced illness. The result is that privately insured patients are able to start treatment earlier in the disease than the publicly insured, and the latter often have no coverage at all.[98]

Insofar as beneficiaries (whether HIV patients or others) substitute Medicaid for more generous private health coverage, the program can reduce the quality of care they receive.

Although policymakers expect that expanding Medicaid and SCHIP will improve the health of low-income families, economists point out there is no evidence that these programs are a cost-effective way of doing so. Economists Helen Levy and David Meltzer write:

> It is clear that expanding health insurance is not the only way to improve health. . . . Policies could also be aimed at factors that may fundamentally contribute to poor health, such as poverty and low levels of education. There is *no evidence* at this time that money aimed at improving health would be better spent on expanding insurance coverage than on any of these other possibilities.[99]

Given that there is no evidence that Medicaid and SCHIP are a cost-effective way of improving health, why are lawmakers so gung-ho to expand these programs? Why does the federal government give states such an enormous financial incentive to expand them?

Reforming Medicaid

To eliminate Medicaid's perverse incentives, the federal government should follow the model provided by the 1996 welfare reform law. That law scaled back federal cash assistance to the poor, and the results were unquestionably positive. Welfare rolls were cut in half and poverty reached the lowest point in a generation. Similarly, the law cut Medicaid benefits for certain immigrants, which resulted in *increased* coverage levels among immigrants.

The now-repealed Aid to Families with Dependent Children cash-assistance program operated like Medicaid in many ways. It conferred a legal entitlement to benefits on anyone who met the eligibility criteria. States received funding from the federal government in the form of an open-ended "match." AFDC was also largely run from Washington, which provided detailed rules on how states should run their programs.

AFDC had been accused of discouraging work and encouraging dependence. The 1996 welfare reform law sought to minimize these incentives by scaling back federal cash assistance for the poor. The federal entitlement to benefits was eliminated; a five-year lifetime limit and work requirements for many recipients were put in its place. Federal funding was frozen and distributed to the states as block grants. This gave states much greater control over benefits, eligibility, and the use of federal funds.

Opponents of the 1996 law predicted that withdrawing assistance in this way would be disastrous for the poor. Some predicted that an additional one million children would be thrown into poverty.[100] Yet withdrawing assistance produced exactly the opposite result. Caseloads plummeted and poverty decreased—often dramatically—for every racial category and age, including children. Although the poverty rate has increased somewhat since 2000, it remained lower in 2005 than at any point in the 17 years leading up to welfare reform.[101] Many who opposed the 1996 law have since admitted that it accomplished a large measure of good.

Medicaid is the forgotten child of welfare reform. In 1995, Congress passed legislation that would have eliminated the federal entitlement to Medicaid benefits, freed states to experiment with different eligibility rules and structures, and converted federal funding from an open-ended "match" to block grants. These changes were vetoed by President Bill Clinton during the budget showdown of 1995. In 1996, Congress dropped such changes from the welfare reform bill in response to a veto threat from President Clinton.

Congress should finish the job of welfare reform by applying its successes to Medicaid. First, Congress should stop encouraging Medicaid expansions and freeze payments to states, just as welfare reform froze payments to states at the 1995 amount. According to Congressional Budget Office figures, freezing federal Medicaid spending at 2007 levels would produce $1.1 trillion in savings by

2017.[102] Second, Congress should give states maximum flexibility to use federal funds to meet a few broad goals, as it did with AFDC's replacement, the Temporary Assistance for Needy Families program. Those goals should include

(1) targeting medical assistance to the truly needy;
(2) reducing dependence;
(3) reducing crowd-out of private effort, including charitable care; and
(4) promoting competitive private markets for medical care and insurance.

A necessary first step toward allowing states to focus resources on the truly needy would be eliminating the federal entitlement to Medicaid benefits, just as Congress eliminated the federal entitlement to cash assistance under TANF.

By themselves, these reforms would not alter a single state's program. Each state would have the power to keep its program running just as it would under current law. In fact, states that want to spend more on their Medicaid programs would be free to do so—and pay for it themselves, rather than force other states to shoulder the burden. However, states likely would experiment with ways of providing efficient care to those who truly need assistance and encouraging private charitable care. As states learn from each others' experiences, they would likely adopt approaches that reduce dependence, health care costs, and the burden Medicaid imposes on taxpayers.

A number of proposed Medicaid reforms would subsidize beneficiaries directly, rather than indirectly when they obtain medical care. These reforms include giving beneficiaries vouchers with which they could purchase private coverage and/or health savings accounts for their out-of-pocket expenses. Some governors, such as Indiana's Mitch Daniels (R), have restructured Medicaid benefits with HSAs. Other states are also considering such proposals.[103] Instead of an open-ended promise of health benefits, beneficiaries would receive money in an HSA to use toward copayments and deductibles, and could keep what they don't spend.

The idea behind vouchers and HSAs is that by giving beneficiaries ownership of their benefits rather than an open-ended subsidy, states would encourage beneficiaries to be prudent consumers and avoid wasteful consumption. This would eliminate administrative costs and help rein in medical inflation to the benefit of all consumers. Allowing Medicaid beneficiaries to manage their health care dollars would also increase Medicaid patients' choice of doctors and force providers to compete to meet the needs of Medicaid patients. These proposals build on what seem to be successful "cash and counseling" programs in Florida, Arkansas, and New Jersey.[104] In these programs, the frail elderly, adults with disabilities, and children with developmental disabilities receive a cash allowance and counseling on how to purchase services directly, rather than have them provided by the state. Beneficiaries get to keep whatever funds they do not spend. Patient satisfaction with such "cash and counseling" programs is high and beneficiaries are able to accumulate some savings through the program, at an overall cost comparable to the previous defined benefits model.[105]

States should experiment with different combinations of in-kind benefits and cash assistance in their Medicaid programs. However, Medicaid HSAs or vouchers may trade one set of problems for another. Beneficiaries should be more careful shoppers if they share in the savings. They would also enjoy greater choice. However, all subsidies increase the incidence of that which is subsidized and become even more attractive the more control they grant the recipient. The very fact that these reforms would give beneficiaries greater control over their benefits may encourage more people to sign up for benefits. Only about two-thirds of Medicaid-eligible individuals are enrolled at any given time,[106] and many do so only for brief periods. A more attractive subsidy could encourage more people to enroll, to stay enrolled for longer periods, and to claim the maximum subsidy. This may have been part of the reason Florida's "cash and counseling" program saw increased outlays in its first year of operation.[107] Thus, moving Medicaid closer to a cash-assistance program could trade lower health care costs for higher Medicaid spending, greater disincentives to work, and more dependence.

This is not to suggest that states should not experiment with vouchers and HSAs. However Medicaid's subsidies are structured, they will create perverse incentives and impose costs on both taxpayers and beneficiaries. States should experiment with different ways of minimizing these perverse incentives and their attendant costs. However, the surest way to minimize them—and the only way to eliminate them—is to minimize or eliminate the subsidy.

Minimizing Medicaid

Scaling back federal cash assistance produced positive results in welfare reform. Would the same be true of Medicaid? A provision of the 1996 welfare reform law suggests the answer is yes. That law contained a little-noticed provision that eliminated Medicaid eligibility for many immigrants. Harvard economist George Borjas examined that provision's effects. He found that Medicaid often attracts recipients who could obtain their own health coverage. Most important, the result of this "draconian" measure was exactly the opposite of what many would predict: coverage among noncitizen immigrants *increased* after they were denied Medicaid benefits.

After this provision went into effect, a number of states responded with programs to preserve coverage for those affected. Borjas examined the coverage rates for affected immigrants with the expectation that "as the Medicaid cutbacks took effect, the proportion of those immigrants covered by some type of health insurance should have declined." To the contrary, he found that "the expected decline in health insurance coverage rates did not materialize. If anything, health insurance coverage rates actually rose slightly in this group." Borjas explains:

> The resolution to this conflicting evidence lies in the fact that the affected immigrants responded to the welfare cutbacks. The immigrants most likely to be adversely affected by the new restrictions significantly increased their labor supply, thereby raising their probability of being covered by employer-sponsored insurance. In fact, this increase in the probability of coverage through employer-sponsored insurance was large enough to completely offset the Medicaid cutbacks. The empirical analysis, therefore, provides strong evidence of a sizable crowd-out effect of publicly provided health insurance among immigrants. *In an important sense, the state programs were unnecessary.* In the absence of these programs, the targeted immigrants themselves would have taken actions to reduce the probability that they would be left without health insurance coverage.[108] (Emphasis added.)

If the state programs designed to protect immigrants from losing coverage were unnecessary, it follows that so too were the original Medicaid subsidies.

The robust economy of the late 1990s cannot explain these results, Borjas argues, because states that offered coverage to those cut from the Medicaid rolls saw coverage levels for this group decrease, while states that did not saw coverage levels increase. Borjas notes that immigrants responded not just to the Medicaid cuts, but to all the changes in the 1996 law. Nonetheless, a natural experiment demonstrated that cutting Medicaid produced results consistent with those of the broader welfare reform, and exactly the opposite of what many would predict. Borjas's research demonstrates that Medicaid requires taxpayers to pay the health care bills of those who could obtain health coverage on their own. And it suggests that the surest way to reduce the costs imposed by Medicaid is to withdraw assistance to those who are most likely to be able to obtain coverage elsewhere. Withdrawing Medicaid assistance need not decrease—and could even increase—coverage levels.

7. Choice and Competition, or Controls?

Health care may be the most intensively regulated sector of the U.S. economy. Government controls the provision of medical care directly by purchasing nearly half of all medical care itself. Through tax laws, it indirectly influences how others purchase medical care. On top of these efforts, thousands of regulations control who can provide medical goods and services, what they can provide, where and how they can provide it, and who can get it.

Regulation can be understood as a form of taxation. Rather than extract wealth from private parties to be spent by government, regulation directs how private actors use private resources. When it limits or prohibits exchanges that would leave all parties better off, regulation denies those parties income and other benefits. Examples include forbidding terminally ill patients to try experimental treatments, or forbidding organ recipients to compensate organ providers and their families. Regulation can also make some exchanges less valuable to one or all parties, such as by requiring health insurance to include coverage that purchasers do not want. When regulation leaves individuals with less income, more risk, or less health, the effect is as harmful as a tax. Health care regulation is often far more harmful, for it can tax one's very life.

Regulatory Costs

Christopher Conover of Duke University recently conducted a first-of-its-kind, comprehensive cost-benefit analysis of health care regulation in the United States.[1] Conover estimated the total social cost of 47 categories of health care regulation. He defines total social cost as "the value of the goods and services lost by society resulting from the use of resources to comply with and implement the regulation, and from reductions in output."[2] Conover estimated that in 2002, health care regulations provided benefits of $170.1 billion. However, the costs outweighed the benefits by a ratio of two to

115

one. Total social costs were $339.2 billion, leaving a net cost of $169.1 billion.

Conover labels the social cost of health care regulations "a $169 billion hidden tax" and offers a number of ways to comprehend its magnitude. Health care regulation costs Americans more than they spend on gasoline and oil ($165.8 billion in 2002) or on pharmaceuticals ($162.4 billion in 2002). "Spread across all households, health services regulation cost the average household an estimated $1,546 in 2002."[3] In fact, the annual cost of health care regulation is 50 percent higher than the fiscal cost of the Iraq war ($109 billion per year).[4] Such regulation makes health insurance unaffordable for an estimated 7.5 million Americans, or one-sixth of those who are uninsured on any given day. Finally, health care regulation reduces societal income and with it society's ability to purchase products that protect lives (e.g., safer homes, safer automobiles). Conover estimates that this effect induces an additional 22,200 deaths per year—4,000 more deaths than the Institute of Medicine estimates are due to Americans lacking health insurance. This figure is also greater than the number of annual deaths from HIV, non-Hodgkin's lymphoma, leukemia, homicide, ovarian cancer, Parkinson's disease, and emphysema. It exceeds the annual number of alcohol-induced deaths (19,344) and is roughly equal to the number of drug-induced deaths (22,296).[5] (See Figure 7.1.)

The cost of health care regulation is equal to roughly 10 percent of all U.S. national health expenditures.[6] It is important to note that Conover's estimate does not include the costs of many other government activities in the health care sector, such as the tax exclusion for employer-provided health benefits (estimated cost: $106 billion in 2002); subsidies that purchase health care of no value (e.g., $34 billion of Medicare spending in 2002) or less value than its cost; or compliance with "continual changes in public payment policies."[7] Including these factors brings the cost of government direction of the health care sector to at least 20 percent of national health expenditures.

Conover does find that some regulations are on balance helpful. In his overall estimate, these net benefits hide part of the cost of the remaining regulations—those that do more harm than good. Taken by itself, this latter group imposes net costs of $204.2 billion annually.[8] It also gives policymakers a good place to begin deregulating America's health care sector.

Figure 7.1
Various Causes of Death (2002)

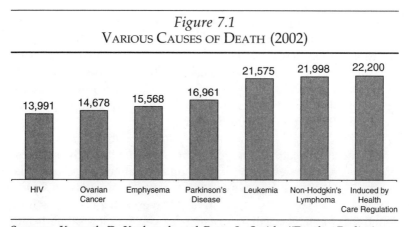

SOURCES: Kenneth D. Kochanek and Betty L. Smith, "Deaths: Preliminary Data for 2002," *National Vital Statistics Reports* (Centers for Disease Control) 52, no. 13 (February 11, 2004): 15–18; and Christopher Conover, "Health Care Regulation: A $169 Billion Hidden Tax," Cato Institute Policy Analysis no. 527, October 4, 2004.

In numerous industries, deregulation has spurred greater consumer choice and competition, which has led to increases in quality and productivity, as well as reduced prices.[9] A consumer-directed health care agenda would deregulate the health care industry to increase competition and give consumers greater freedom of choice, including the ability to choose the level of regulatory and legal protection they desire.

Choice and Competition in Health Insurance

State and federal governments have enacted layers of regulation that place restrictions on the pricing, composition, administration, and cancellation of health insurance policies. Regulations that restrict insurers' ability to offer and price health insurance according to risk force low-risk customers to subsidize high-risk customers, and price low-risk and low-income consumers out of the market.

Many health insurance regulations are meant to correct the unintended consequences of other laws and regulations. Such regulations include those laws that require employers to provide health benefits to former employees, as well as those that require insurers to cover services from providers that may otherwise be excluded from coverage. In many cases, health care regulations are an attempt by private

117

interests to seek private gain. For example, states have enacted an estimated 1,823 separate benefit mandates that require health insurers to cover particular services, including "acupuncture, massage therapists and hair prostheses (wigs)."[10] The most vocal proponents of laws requiring consumers to purchase acupuncture, massage therapy, and chiropractic coverage are (not surprisingly) acupuncturists, massage therapists, and chiropractors.

The costs of health insurance regulation are substantial. Conover finds that some health insurance regulations yield benefits in excess of their costs. However, the remaining regulations impose annual costs of $46.6 billion in excess of the benefits they provide.[11] Grace-Marie Arnett (Turner) and Melinda Schriver of the Galen Institute found that the 16 states that most aggressively regulated their health insurance markets in the 1990s saw their uninsured populations grow eight times faster than other states.[12] The FTC cautions legislators on the harms of benefit mandates:

> Governments should reconsider whether current mandates best serve their citizens' health care needs. When deciding whether to mandate particular benefits, governments should consider that such mandates are likely to reduce competition, restrict consumer choice, raise the cost of health insurance, and increase the number of uninsured Americans.[13]

Some states already see the wisdom of deregulation. After leading the trend toward greater regulation in the 1990s, officials in Maryland are attempting to relax expensive mandated benefits.[14] Excessive regulation in Kentucky drove 45 health insurance companies out of the state, dramatically increased health premiums, and increased the number of uninsured Kentuckians by 17 percent in 8 years. Legislators have begun to deregulate that state's health insurance market. Liberalized prices and other reforms have brought five insurers back to the state and are giving Kentuckians more choices.[15] New Hampshire enacted price controls and other regulations in 1994. By 1997, its insurance commissioner reported, "the quality of products available in this market is worsening . . . the cost of available products in this market is increasing . . . [and] the loss ratios of the writing carriers [have] increased." In 2002, New Hampshire lawmakers relaxed price controls. At least two carriers have returned to the state.[16]

Interstate Commerce in Health Insurance

The same competitive process that drives producers to improve quality and reduce costs can help produce higher-quality regulation. The federal and state governments should allow health insurance purchasers to choose the state that regulates their coverage. Competition among states would lead them to tailor their regulatory regimes to consumers' preferences and to abandon regulations that make health coverage unappealing or too costly.

Currently, health insurance purchasers are largely stuck with the regulatory regime of the state where they reside.[17] If free to choose health insurance policies regulated by states other than their own, consumers could avoid regulations that impose unwanted costs. Instead, they could "purchase" another state's set of regulations by purchasing coverage from an insurer chartered in that state. If Minnesotans do not want to purchase all 60 types of coverage mandated there, they could choose to purchase health insurance regulated by Idaho, which has the fewest mandated benefits (13), or by another state whose laws are aligned more closely with their preferences. In addition to mandated benefits, consumers could avoid price controls and other unwanted regulations.

Insurers would advertise either the types of regulatory protections that accompany a particular policy, or the state that regulates it. Rating agencies such as *Consumer Reports* could publicize the strengths and weaknesses of each state's set of laws. Branding— for example, "Licensed in Minnesota"—would earn each state a reputation for being consumer-friendly, too lax, or too onerous.

Many purchasers would choose less regulation. For example, low-risk and low-income consumers might opt for coverage that does not force them to subsidize high-risk and higher-income consumers. Others would prefer greater regulatory protections. The cost of those protections would be reflected in a policy's premiums, and consumers could then decide whether the increased protections are worth the price.

Millions of Americans shopping online and offline in a nationwide market for health insurance would put enormous pressure on states to deregulate. Each state's interest in premium tax revenue, and having insurers domicile in their state, would encourage competition among states to provide the protections consumers want while keeping health insurance affordable. States currently compete for the business of firms and investors in a similar market for corporate chartering laws. Delaware has taken a dominant position in this market by offering a set of laws that satisfy its customers. There is no reason Delaware or another state could not do the same with health insurance regulation.

The federal government should give all Americans the right to purchase health insurance regulated by the state of their choice. One survey found 72 percent of likely voters support allowing consumers to purchase health insurance from another state.[18] Rep. John Shadegg (R-Ariz.) has introduced legislation that would facilitate purchasing health insurance across state lines.[19] That legislation would allow consumers in the individual market to avoid costly benefit mandates in their own states. However, there is no reason to limit such choice to individual consumers or to benefit mandates. Shadegg's legislation should be expanded to include employers and other group purchasers, and additional types of regulation. States can give their own residents this right without waiting for Congress to act.

Efforts to liberalize or repeal discrete regulations are useful. However, consumers would be better off if lawmakers put deregulation on autopilot by allowing competition to find an equilibrium between too much and too little regulation.

Can Competition Improve Medical Technology Regulation?

> *The Newtonian principle of gravitation is now more firmly established, on the basis of reason, than it would be were the government to step in, and to make it an article of necessary faith. Reason and experiment have been indulged, and error has fled before them . . . Subject opinion to coercion: whom will you make your inquisitors? Fallible men; men governed by bad passions, by private as well as public reasons.*
>
> —Thomas Jefferson, *Notes on the State of Virginia*,
> 1781–1785[20]

Another area of regulation that imposes costs in excess of its benefits is regulation of pharmaceuticals and medical devices. In an attempt to ensure that such products are safe and effective, the federal government prohibits patients and doctors from using any such products that have not completed the U.S. Food and Drug Administration's lengthy approval process. The power to withhold new drugs and medical devices from even terminally ill patients gives the FDA a monopoly over the initial safety and efficacy certification of such products.

Rigorous testing of pharmaceuticals and medical devices often provides crucial information. But is a single government monopoly the best system for protecting the public against the dual threats of unsafe medical products and delayed access to innovative, life-saving treatments? Despite the good intentions of the FDA and its supporters, evidence suggests that its monopoly increases morbidity and mortality. Lifting the FDA's monopoly would restore the freedom of patients to choose their own course of medical treatment. In its place, private accreditation agencies and the courts would ensure that medical products are thoroughly tested. Moreover, those institutions would remove unsafe products from the market, just as they do today.

The FDA vs. Patient's Rights

The FDA's power to withhold new treatments is a threat to the freedom and the health of patients. Each year, the agency denies terminally ill patients access to experimental treatments that might improve or save their lives. One such patient was Abigail Burroughs, a college student who was diagnosed with head and neck cancer in 2001. Abigail has been described as "[t]he very picture of idealism and promise—an honor-roll achiever at the University of Virginia who tutored needy school kids and volunteered at a homeless shelter."[21]

Abigail soon exhausted all available therapies in her battle against cancer. On the advice of her oncologist, Abigail attempted to obtain the then-unapproved cancer drugs Iressa and Erbitux through the few channels allowed by the FDA. Abigail's father, Frank Burroughs, testified to Congress, "We tried to get Abigail into narrowly defined clinical trials, but she did not qualify for them. We worked very hard to acquire the drugs on a compassionate basis and got nowhere."[22] Abigail died in June 2001. The FDA approved Iressa in 2003 and Erbitux in 2004. Although the FDA approved Erbitux for colorectal cancer, the drug has since shown promise in fighting head and neck cancers.[23] A senior FDA official later commented on terminally ill patients' access to experimental drugs, "In general, I think that what exists is sufficient."[24]

It cannot be known whether Iressa or Erbitux would have lengthened Abigail Burroughs' life. However, it is clear that Congress, through the FDA, denied Abigail the right to choose her own course of medical treatment. Shortly after Abigail's death, Frank Burroughs founded the nonprofit Abigail Alliance for Better Access to Developmental Drugs with other terminally ill patients and their survivors. The group helps terminally ill patients obtain experimental treatments through existing channels. It has also filed suit against the FDA for violating "the constitutional privacy and liberty rights of terminally ill patients, including numerous Abigail Alliance members, and their constitutional guarantee against deprivation of life without due process."[25]

Abigail Burroughs' story is just one example of how FDA regulation denies patients their freedom to choose their course of treatment and the benefits of new therapies. FDA regulation also prevents the introduction of many therapies, delays the introduction of others, increases their cost once they become available, and limits the spread of information about new discoveries.

The Costs of FDA Regulation

The time and expense required to gain FDA approval of a new drug has grown enormously in recent decades. The number of years required to shepherd a new drug through the FDA's approval process nearly doubled from 8.1 years in the 1960s to 15.2 years in the 1990s.[26] The monetary cost of new drug approval has grown even more rapidly. In the *Journal of Health Economics*, Joseph DiMasi, Ronald Hansen, and Henry Grabowski estimate the cost of bringing a new drug to patients has doubled since 1987 to more than $800 million, while a new drug discovered in 2003 will cost $1.9 billion to bring to patients by 2015.[27] Texas A&M University economist Steven Wiggins estimated that by the 1970s, the growing cost of FDA regulation reduced the number of new drugs introduced annually in the United States by 60 percent.[28] The growing monetary cost of the approval process, coupled with reduced price competition from having fewer drugs approved, increases the price of drugs that do reach patients.

The longer the FDA's drug approval process, the more patients endure illness or die waiting for the agency to approve new drug therapies. The *Washington Post* editorializes, "As hundreds of

Figure 7.2
FDA Regulation: Lives Saved vs. Lives Lost

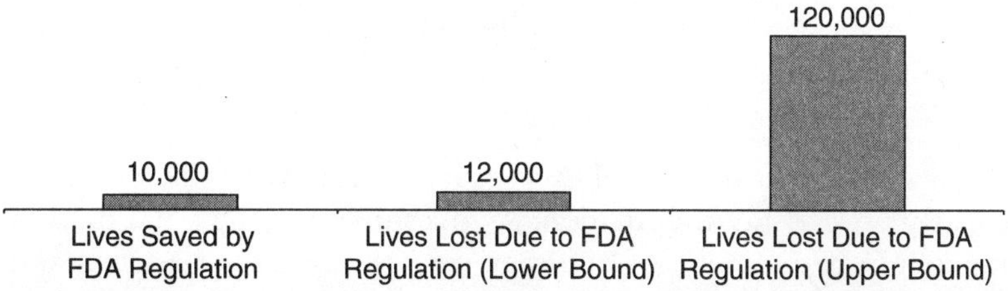

Source: Dale H. Gieringer, "The Safety and Efficacy of New Drug Approval," *Cato Journal* 5, no. 1 (Spring/Summer 1985): 177–201.

patients' groups can attest, there are high costs when the FDA does not approve drugs quickly, even drugs with serious side effects. People die every day waiting for new treatments."[29] Studies have estimated that the FDA's delays in approving such drugs as Misoprostol (ulcers) and beta blockers (heart attacks) resulted in tens of thousands of unnecessary deaths by patients who could have been saved by the drugs.[30]

Finally, once a drug is approved, the FDA prevents manufacturers from advertising new uses for it, even if those uses have been proven by rigorous scientific testing and promoted by medical journals and other experts. In one notorious example, for years the FDA prevented aspirin manufacturers from advertising the drug's ability to save lives following a heart attack. The FDA's censorship of the benefits of just one drug's ability to fight just one medical condition may have resulted in as many as 40,000 to 80,000 preventable deaths.[31]

Without a doubt, FDA regulation has kept unsafe drugs off the market. Yet it has also kept beneficial drugs off the market as well. Many of these have been treatments the FDA has rendered uneconomical to pursue. Drugs that treat rare diseases with small patient populations make recouping the costs of drug approval impossible. Moreover, the lives FDA regulation has saved by blocking unsafe drugs are far outweighed by the lives lost due to its suppression of beneficial drugs. While a policy consultant with the Decisions and Ethics Center of the Department of Engineering-Economic Systems at Stanford University, Dale Gieringer estimated that FDA regulation results in anywhere from 21,000 to 120,000 lives lost per decade, yet prevents at most 10,000 deaths from unsafe drugs[32] (see Figure 7.2). Indeed, the handful of studies that have attempted to quantify the costs and benefits of FDA drug regulation have unanimously concluded that the marginal costs of such regulation exceed the marginal benefits.[33] Conover monetizes the net cost of FDA regulation at $42 billion annually.[34]

Biased toward Delay

The growing cost of the FDA's approval processes is an inevitable consequence of FDA regulation. A government agency that holds a monopoly over safety and efficacy certification of new drugs and medical devices will always favor more testing and greater delay, even at the cost of patient freedom and lost lives. The reason stems from how the public responds to the two different kinds of mistakes that the FDA can make.

The first type of mistake, known as a "Type I error," occurs when the FDA approves a drug that turns out to be harmful. When this happens, those patients who are injured are easily identified, and the public intuitively links the injury to the FDA's error. The second type of mistake is called a "Type II error." These occur when the agency rejects or delays approval of a beneficial product, preventing the product from reaching patients.

Although both types of errors result in unnecessary pain or death, the public responds differently to Type I and Type II errors, which in turn affects how the FDA seeks to avoid them. When the FDA approves a drug that can harm people (a Type I error), the victims are easily identifiable. Those who are harmed by the drug are thrust before the public eye. They (or their survivors) can appear on the news and testify before Congress. As a result, Type I errors subject agency officials to congressional investigations, public reproach, professional humiliation, and unemployment. In contrast, victims of Type II errors are largely invisible. When the FDA delays or rejects approval of a beneficial drug, it is axiomatic that the FDA's error will permit continued suffering and avoidable deaths. However, the harm is attributed to the underlying illness, such as cancer or heart disease, rather than to the FDA's error. As a result, victims of Type II errors are much harder to identify, even if their numbers are greater.[35]

Because Type II errors typically leave few fingerprints, FDA officials have a personal incentive to minimize Type I errors, even at the cost of committing more Type II errors. As a former FDA commissioner observed:

> Wherever a controversy over a new drug is resolved by its
> approval the Agency and the individuals involved likely will
> be investigated. Whenever such a drug is disapproved, no
> inquiry will be made.[36]

Although the agency receives the full measure of criticism when a patient dies from a Type I error, it receives relatively little criticism when patients die from Type II errors. Put another way, the FDA doesn't bear its full share of the blame for Type II errors.

Given these incentives, the FDA understandably attempts to minimize Type I errors, even at the cost of more Type II errors. The primary way it does so is to increase the length and expense of the approval process. For example, increasing the number, duration, and size of the clinical trials required for approval gives the agency more time and information to eliminate Type I errors. However, it accomplishes this at the expense of a longer and more costly approval process, which increases Type II errors. Institutionally, the agency is predisposed toward delay and more costly approvals. Dr. Henry Miller, another former FDA official, explains how these incentives operate in practice:

> In the early 1980s, when I headed the team at the FDA that
> was reviewing the [new drug application] for recombinant
> human insulin, the first drug made with gene-splicing tech-
> niques, we were ready to recommend approval a mere four
> months after the application was submitted (at a time when
> the average time for NDA review was more than two and
> a half years) . . . [M]y supervisor refused to sign off on the
> approval—even though he agreed that the data provided
> compelling evidence of the drug's safety and effectiveness.
> "If anything goes wrong," he argued, "think how bad it
> will look that we approved the drug so quickly" . . . The
> supervisor was more concerned with not looking bad in case
> of an unforeseen mishap than with getting an important new
> product to patients who needed it.[37]

As noted earlier, the duration of the FDA's new drug approval process has doubled since the 1960s, and the financial cost has doubled since the late 1980s. In addition, from 1977 to 1995, the number of clinical trials required for each new drug doubled and the number of patients involved in those trials nearly tripled.[38] In 1992 and again in 1997, Congress authorized the FDA to collect "user fees" from drug manufacturers. These additional resources enabled the agency to hire more staff and have shortened review times for new drug applications. However, the lion's share of the new drug approval process is devoted to testing; the year or so dedicated to FDA review of a new drug application is the last and shortest part of the new drug approval process.[39] It is uncertain whether shorter review times have affected the growth in overall approval time—the time from synthesis of a new drug until it is made available to patients. The available data on the growing monetary cost of the approval process and the growth in clinical trials are not encouraging.

Expanding access to safe, effective, and affordable drugs and medical devices cannot be achieved by reforms that tinker with the FDA, such as charging applicants user fees for product approval. It requires lifting the FDA's monopoly and restoring the freedom of individuals to make their own medical decisions.

Competitive Regulation of Medical Technology

A model for FDA reform exists in the private sector. The United States already has a nongovernment, market-based system that certifies the effectiveness of drugs and medical devices.[40] This private system begins to work after the FDA approves a new product. For example, when the agency approves a drug for a particular use, that approved use goes on the drug's label. However, physicians may and often do prescribe the drug for other uses. Using the pain reliever aspirin to fight heart attacks is one example of an "off-label" use. Although Viagra was intended as a treatment for angina, it was later found to remedy erectile dysfunction, and has been used to treat pulmonary hypertension, including in premature babies. Had Erbitux been approved in time, Abigail Burroughs' oncologist could have prescribed it off-label for her head and neck cancer, even though the drug had been approved for colorectal cancer.

Lack of FDA certification does not mean such uses are dangerous, untested, or unproven. Off-label uses are suggested or discovered by doctors and scientists, tested, and discussed worldwide in medical journals and symposia. If validated, they appear in medical textbooks, the *U.S. Pharmacopoeia Drug Information* (*USP*), the *American Hospital Formulary Service Drug Information*, and other authoritative resources. In fact, off-label uses often become the standard of care, particularly in fighting cancer and other diseases. Doctors so frequently rely on market-based certification (which arguably includes foreign governments' certifications), that over half of known drug uses are off-label uses.

Coupled with the tort system, private safety and efficacy certification often beats the FDA at its own game. While testing the pain reliever Vioxx for an off-label use, scientists discovered a safety risk (a higher incidence of heart attacks) that FDA reviewers had missed. In 2004, Merck withdrew Vioxx from the market. The pursuit of informal, private certification of an off-label use revealed a risk that FDA regulation had not. The threat of litigation forced Merck to pull the drug from the market. The episode demonstrates that private certification and the tort system can and already do protect patients from unsafe drugs. Market-based certification is also more efficient than the FDA. One study found that off-label uses that were later certified by the FDA were certified by the market (in the *USP*) an average of 2.5 years sooner.[41]

Today's market-based system of private, competitive, off-label certifications respects the freedom of doctors and patients to make treatment decisions according to individual circumstances. The federal government should build on this success and allow companies to seek initial safety and efficacy certification of drugs and medical devices from medical journals (e.g., the *Journal of the American Medical Association*, the *New England Journal of Medicine*), medical schools and textbooks, the *USP*, the *American Hospital Formulary Service Drug Information*, and so forth. These organizations would certify new uses of *new* drugs and medical devices, just as they now certify new uses of *existing* drugs and devices. They would design and execute the laboratory tests and human studies appropriate for evaluating the safety and efficacy of even drugs tailored to individual patients.

To survive in the market, private certification agencies would have to be scrupulously honest: just as Underwriters Laboratories and *Consumer Reports* sell their reputations, the *USP* or other organizations would sell their reputations and lose customers if their reputations came into question. After Vioxx was recalled, critics alleged the FDA took too long to act either because the agency is too cozy with drug manufacturers or too reluctant to admit a mistake. Many have called for an agency independent of the FDA to monitor the safety of drugs after they are introduced and "to second-guess the decisions of the officials who approved the drug in the first place."[42] Private certification already does just that. Medical journals second-guess each other's work in the pursuit of science, prestige, and market share. They and other private accreditors would second-guess each other's work (and their own) because each would profit from building a reputation as being the most honest and scientifically rigorous body. Private accreditation could also take over other duties of the FDA, including monitoring manufacturing processes, product advertisements, and post-market safety.

A competitive system of private certification holds a significant safety advantage over the current FDA monopoly. First, like the FDA, private accreditors would minimize Type I errors to avoid liability and preserve their reputations. However, unlike the FDA, private certification would also minimize Type II errors. The key is competition. In a competitive market, private accreditors would compete for the confidence of doctors and patients and the business of drug manufacturers—on the basis of not only rigorous oversight, but efficiency as well. Those that require unnecessary testing or that needlessly delay certification decisions would lose business to competitors who offer an equally rigorous review at a lower cost. The manufacturer's desire for an efficient certification process could act as a proxy for the patient's need to be protected from unnecessary delay (i.e., Type II errors). Because it enjoys a monopoly position, the FDA is insulated from such pressures and can impose unnecessary costs without fear. In contrast, private certification would protect patients from both Type I and Type II errors. Moreover, Type II errors would be less prevalent under a regime of private certification if only because private accreditors cannot prevent patients from obtaining an unapproved drug.

As discussed in Chapter 1, the benefits of pharmaceutical innovations often overwhelm the costs. Indeed, new drug therapies even reduce spending on hospitalization and other areas of care. The FDA's power to overrule the choices of patients and their doctors, plus the agency's monopoly over the approval of new medical technologies, unnecessarily hamper the pursuit of new technologies and make patients less safe. Restoring patients' freedom to use any non-FDA approved product and allowing private organizations and the courts to regulate medical treatments would help Americans capture the benefits of future pharmaceutical innovations that the current FDA certification process is likely to suppress.

What to Do about the Shortage of Transplantable Organs

The year 2004 marked the 50th anniversary of the first successful human organ transplant, in which doctors transplanted a kidney from a man into his twin brother. At that time and for some time thereafter, there was no shortage of transplantable organs. The ability to perform transplants was rare and the technology limited to transplants between close, living relatives. Because the first suppliers were relatives and transplants were rare, altruistic organ donation was sufficient to meet demand.

As transplant technology advanced and diffused, however, more doctors became able to transplant more organs from more donors into more recipients. Demand for transplantable organs grew. The development of immunosuppressive drugs enabled transplants from cadavers, which greatly increased the number of patients considered candidates for organ transplants.

Yet relying solely on altruistic donation meant that the supply of organs stagnated, and queues began to form. When one doctor attempted to increase the supply through payments to live kidney donors, Congress reacted by passing the 1984 National Organ Transplant Act. That act made it a felony to offer financial incentives to potential organ providers. Since then, technology has continued to expand what medicine can accomplish with transplantation, but the supply of transplantable organs has remained stagnant. Before long, waiting lists began to form.

The United Network for Organ Sharing is the nonprofit organization that contracts with the federal government to manage the waiting lists. UNOS reports that almost 29,000 Americans received organ transplants in 2006, thanks to 14,757 donors. Yet even this record number of donors could not meet the need. More than 48,000 candidates were added to the waiting lists that year. Those waiting for organs outnumber donors by six to one. By June 2007, the waiting list reached more than 96,000 patients, and another name is added to the waiting lists every 11 minutes[43] (see Figure 7.3).

As a result, more than 6,000 patients died while on the waiting lists in 2006—one every 86 minutes.[44] Although some of these deaths cannot be attributed to the shortage of organs, death is not the only

Figure 7.3
TRANSPLANTABLE ORGANS: THE GROWING GULF BETWEEN
DEMAND AND SUPPLY

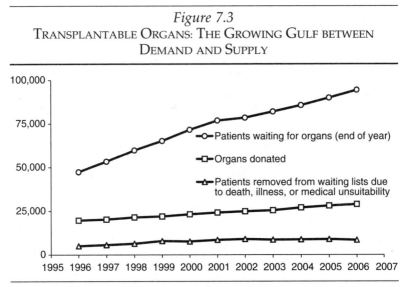

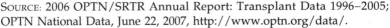

SOURCE: 2006 OPTN/SRTR Annual Report: Transplant Data 1996–2005; OPTN National Data, June 22, 2007, http://www.optn.org/data/.

measure of harm caused by the shortage. Shortages lead to more stringent criteria for admission to the waiting lists, causing many potential transplant candidates to be kept off the lists entirely. As those on the lists wait, they endure significant suffering and expense. Their conditions deteriorate, some to the point that the long-awaited transplant is less successful than it could have been. Thousands deteriorate until they no longer are good candidates for transplantation, and are removed from the list. In 2006, 2,294 patients were removed from the waiting lists because they were "medically unsuitable" or had become "too sick to transplant."[45] Many die soon afterward.

Altruistic organ donation may have been enough to satisfy the demand for transplantable organs in a time of primitive technology. It is inadequate today, and will be even more so as transplant technology continues to advance. Previous attempts to meet the growing demand for transplantable organs, such as more funding for education campaigns, have failed. It is clear that the National Organ Transplant Act is an obstacle to satisfying the demand for transplantable organs. A consensus is emerging that something new must be tried, and that something should include markets.

Eliminating a Manmade Shortage

There is no actual shortage of transplantable organs. Economists David Kaserman and A. H. Barnett estimate that each year enough Americans die under conditions that make their organs suitable for transplant to meet the entire demand. Yet most of these organs are buried with the deceased rather than harvested to help the living. Instead of an actual shortage of organs, there exists an *artificial* shortage created by the prohibition of payments for transplantable organs.

That prohibition is effectively a price control that sets the price of transplantable organs at zero dollars in spite of the immense value they hold. Because government prevents the price from rising above $0, it effectively hides from potential providers information about the great need for transplantable organs. In 2000, 539 economists signed an open letter on health care reform that explained the dynamics of such price controls: "For thousands of years, governments have tried to control prices. The universal experience has been that price controls produce shortages . . ."[46] With Congress having written into law that transplantable organs have zero value, it should come as no surprise that so many Americans act as if that were the case.

Kaserman and Barnett estimate that lifting the prohibition with regard to organs from cadavers would eliminate the artificial shortage and the waiting lists. They estimate that payments would be substantially lower than $1,000 per organ. That is a relatively modest sum compared with the monetary and pain-and-suffering costs associated with waiting for organs. Considering the amounts now spent to encourage donation, Kaserman and Barnett posit, "It is entirely possible that we are now spending more to elicit 'free' donations than it would cost to purchase organs."[47]

Allowing payments to organ providers would convey the human need that government price controls currently hide. Payments would be negotiated by recipients and providers and could go to the decedent's family or could be donated to charities according to the decedent's will. With procedural controls and penalties sufficiently harsh to ensure that all exchanges are truly consensual, such a reform could encompass payments to living organ providers. Congress could eliminate America's manmade organ shortage by repealing or amending the National Organ Transplant Act to allow such payments. At a minimum, Congress should allow payments for cadaveric organs.

Is Paying for Organs Ethical?

This reform no doubt raises ethical considerations. In 2004, Congress directed the Secretary of Health and Human Services to study the ethical implications of using financial incentives to increase cadaveric "donations." The request originally came from Senate Majority Leader Bill Frist (R-Tenn.), himself a transplant surgeon. Such an examination must address the ethical implications of the prohibition on payments and the resulting shortage. Is it ethical to force thousands of patients to suffer and die for an ethos they may not share? What are the ethical implications of allowing the state to control what free individuals may do with their own bodies?

A leading ethical objection to organ payments is that it would be inegalitarian: lifting the ban could lead to a situation where mostly poor individuals sell their organs to the rich. That seems to occur in the international market for live kidneys.[48] One way to allay this objection would be to allow payments only for cadaveric organs. Doing so would decrease the demand for live organs that fuels an international black market.

What also might allay such concerns is the result of such transactions. When a wealthy recipient purchases a kidney from a poor provider, the result is *two living human beings*. All too often, the alternative is *one living and one dead human being*.[49]

Many suppose that the current prohibition is more egalitarian because wealthy transplant patients would more often face the possibility of death on a waiting list. Yet America's manmade organ shortage is also highly inegalitarian, favoring the rich at the expense of the poor. While tens of thousands of Americans wait years and often die waiting for organs, celebrities like Mickey Mantle jump to the head of the waiting lists.[50] Basketball star Alonzo Mourning's fame induced more than 500 people to offer him one of their kidneys. Yet patients without fame are forbidden to use what resources they do possess (e.g., health insurance) to save their own lives or the lives of their loved ones.

America's manmade shortage also disproportionately harms minorities. Blacks account for 12 percent of the U.S. population and

Figure 7.4
AFRICAN-AMERICANS: SHARE OF U.S. POPULATION AND SHARE
OF PATIENTS WAITING FOR ORGANS

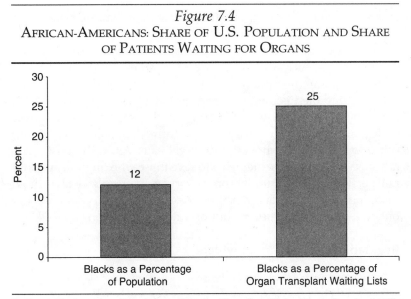

SOURCE: Christopher Windham, "Blacks Urged to Help Close Gap in Availability of Donor Organs," *Wall Street Journal*, November 24, 2004, p. D4.

a comparable share of organ donors. Yet blacks account for 25 percent of those waiting for an organ[51] (see Figure 7.4).

Forcing the Issue

Lloyd Cohen of George Mason University has chosen a novel way to highlight the ethical objections to the ban on organ payments.[52] Cohen has executed legal documents that give permission for his organs to be harvested under only two conditions. The first is that the organ go to a family member or a member in good standing of the LifeSharers organization.[53] Otherwise, Cohen denies permission for his organs to be harvested unless his estate is paid $864.27 per organ.[54] If his estate is not paid, his organs will perish.

Cohen's goal is not to be a curmudgeon, but to illuminate the choice that opponents of organ payments have made for themselves and for others. When Cohen dies, those who oppose payments will face two options: (1) violate their principles and pay up, or (2) allow yet another patient to die unnecessarily. Those who choose the latter, Cohen writes, "must hold that it is morally preferable, because it celebrates 'the intrinsic ineliminable, ineluctable value of human life

133

and health,' that a 12-year-old girl die from liver failure rather than that the organ that would save her life be provided by a market."[55] Cohen encourages others to give similar directions for the disposition of their organs. As more people do so, he argues, it will force society to recognize the unethical choice that is being forced on us.

Respecting the freedom of organ providers and recipients would eliminate the artificial organ shortage and save thousands of lives each year. As more transplants are performed, new discoveries will cause technological innovation to accelerate. As in the past, such advances would enable medicine to save those who previously could not be helped. The prohibition on organ payments delays those discoveries and retards innovation. As a result, it imposes costs not only on current generations, but on future generations as well.

Regulating Health Care Providers

> *The State stands a Gibraltar between me and anybody who insists upon prescribing for my soul what I don't want to take . . . why shouldn't I have equal liberty with regard to my body, which is of so much less concern? . . . I don't know that I cared much about these osteopaths until I heard you were going to drive them out of the State; but since I heard this I haven't been able to sleep . . . Now what I contend is that my body is my own, at least I have always so regarded it. If I do harm through my experimenting with it, it is I who suffer, not the State.*
>
> —Mark Twain[56]

Regulation can be used as a tool for crippling one's competitors. This is most evident in regulations that bar individuals from entering a profession or providing certain services. The moratorium on the creation or expansion of specialty hospitals discussed earlier is one example. States also have enacted numerous laws that restrict who may provide health care services. Such laws restrict the freedom of individuals to choose their profession and their health care providers. As such, the burden of demonstrating that barriers to entry into health care markets result in better health outcomes falls on supporters. Not only have supporters failed to meet this burden, but persuasive evidence suggests such barriers increase health care costs and have either no effect or a negative effect on health care quality.

Competition among Health Professionals

To practice medicine in the United States, medical professionals typically must obtain a state license. In addition to restricting entry into the medical professions, licensing laws also prohibit some providers from providing certain services, require others to practice in particular settings, and act as a barrier to competition from providers with identical licenses from another state. As the FTC explains, "State licensing boards composed primarily of physicians determine, apply, and enforce the requirements for physicians to practice within a particular state. Various state licensing boards have taken steps to restrict 'allied health professionals' and telemedicine. Some states have limited or no reciprocity for licensing physicians and allied health professionals already licensed by another state."[57]

Allied health professionals include nonphysician medical workers such as dental hygienists, diagnostic medical sonographers, dietitians, medical technicians, nurse midwives, nurse anesthetists, nurse practitioners, occupational therapists, physical therapists, physician assistants, psychologists, radiographers, respiratory therapists, and speech language pathologists. Such practitioners often provide services comparable to what physicians provide, but at the same or lower cost. Studies have shown that within the scope of their training, nurse practitioners perform comparably to physicians in terms of cost, health outcomes, and patient satisfaction.[58] Nonetheless, many states' licensing laws forbid allied health professionals from having direct access to patients and prohibit these professionals from opening independent practices.

Licensing also restricts the freedom of physicians by limiting their ability to practice in states where there is a need. Most states restrict the practice of telemedicine, often requiring already licensed out-of-state physicians to obtain an additional license. The FTC writes, "Studies consistently have found that state-based licensure can harm consumer welfare by serving as a barrier to provider mobility."[59]

The Cost of Licensing

Despite the fact that occupational licensing affects a larger portion of the labor market than either the minimum wage or unionization laws, it has received less attention from academics, particularly in recent years.[60] Nonetheless, a number of studies demonstrate that licensing laws reduce the availability of medical care and increase its

135

Figure 7.5
Cost of Medical Licensure vs. Added Income to Licensed Professionals

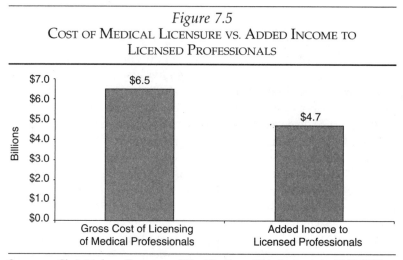

Sources: Christopher Conover, "Health Care Regulation: A $169 Billion Hidden Tax," Cato Institute Policy Analysis no. 527, October 4, 2004.

cost.[61] In his Pulitzer Prize–winning history of American medicine, Princeton University sociologist Paul Starr quotes former American Medical Association president William Allan Pusey on the impact of licensing doctors:

> As you increase the cost of the license to practice medicine you increase the price at which medical service must be sold and you correspondingly decrease the number of people who can afford to buy this medical service.[62]

Conover estimates that licensing of medical professionals costs Americans $6.5 billion per year, $4.7 billion of which is channeled to licensed professionals in the form of higher incomes[63] (see Figure 7.5). That is largely the purpose of such laws. In a 1984 study, economist Chris W. Paul found that "licensing legislation was the result of organized physicians employing the political system for limiting entry and the concomitant increasing of return to incumbent medical practitioners."[64]

The lack of competition resulting from licensing and scope-of-practice rules has left many without affordable access to medical care. A 2002 survey found that nearly six million Americans turned to alternative medicine (e.g., herbal remedies) to treat illnesses like chronic pain or depression because traditional medical care was too expensive.[65] "Indeed, the creation and development of nurse practitioners (NPs) and physician assistants (PAs)," wrote Congress' Office of Technology Assessment in 1986, "occurred in large part in response to the limited accessibility of basic medical services, especially in rural and inner-city areas, where physicians were disinclined to practice." However, "Legislation and regulations . . . generally tie medical practice by NPs, PAs, and, to some extent, [certified nurse midwives] to associations with physicians and limit such practice where physicians are not present."[66]

Does Licensing Improve Quality of Care?

Supporters claim that the quality of medical care would suffer if not for government licensing requirements, which ensure high-quality practitioners through both rigorous testing and peer oversight. Data regarding the effect of licensing on the quality of medical care are scant. What data do exist, however, suggest it is more likely that public health suffers under compulsory licensing of medical professionals because fewer individuals are able to afford medical care.

In 1989, the federally chartered Institute of Medicine expressed skepticism about the effect of medical licensure on health care access and quality: "It appears that widespread use of licensure carries with it higher costs to consumers [and] reduced access to health care services . . . Although these control mechanisms are designed and carried out in the stated interest of protecting the health and welfare of the public, their effectiveness in this regard has been mixed at best."[67] Similarly, Indiana State University professor Stanley Gross surveyed the academic literature on the quality effects of licensing across numerous occupations in 1986. He noted that

> There is some support for the proposition that entry restrictions result in more qualified professionals to serve the public, as judged by the somewhat questionable ratings of peers, the self-reports of professionals themselves, and crude measures of consumer satisfaction (reduced malpractice claims and rates). However, measures of quality that tap the availability of professional services, the extent to which consumers choose to substitute other practitioners, and the direct outcomes of service primarily show either no relationship between entry restrictions and quality or a negative relationship.[68]

Gross found claims that licensing bodies police the quality of work by their charges even less plausible:

> It has been shown that licensing boards do not effectively determine initial competence of licensees; they do not help to maintain the continued competence of licensees; they are ineffective in the disciplining of errant practitioners; and they do not properly address the needs of underserved populations. Instead, as has been shown, the licensing system has exacerbated the problems of maldistribution and underutilization of professionals, and it has supported a "licensing for life" system.[69]

Compulsory licensing of medical professionals makes health care markets less flexible and less able to respond to patient demand. It also relieves existing professionals of the burden of having to compete with new health care providers and novel ways that others might deliver care to patients. Because it increases the cost of medical education, decreases the supply of providers, and hampers competition, licensure increases health care costs to the detriment of the poorest patients. As a result, many forgo medical care entirely, obtain treatment that is too little or too late, or turn to less expensive (and often more risky) forms of treatment. One extreme example is people who have attempted at-home root canals to avoid the expense of going to the dentist.[70]

In 1962, Milton Friedman wrote, "I am myself persuaded that licensure has reduced both the quantity and the quality of medical practice; that it has reduced the opportunities available to people who would like to be physicians, forcing them to pursue occupations they regard as less attractive; that it has forced the public to pay more for less satisfactory medical service, and that it has retarded technological development both in medicine itself and in the organization of medical practice. I conclude that licensure should be eliminated as a requirement for the practice of medicine."[71]

Reforming Medical Licensure

Reducing harmful government barriers to greater competition in the practice of medicine would benefit patients and many medical professionals. The FTC recommends that states "decrease barriers to entry into provider markets."[72] Reformers typically look to two alternatives for liberalizing licensure laws.

The first is to move from licensure to a system of government certification. State or quasi-governmental bodies (like today's licensing boards) would establish criteria for the initial and continued certification of individuals as competent to practice a particular area. However, providers would be free to practice without certification. Although patients would be free to obtain treatment from the providers of their choice, they would be very cautious about noncertified providers. Certification exists today for nurse midwives as well as physicians who voluntarily choose to become board-certified in a particular specialty.

The second option is referred to as registration, whereby providers may practice medicine simply by registering their practice with the state, in other words, without having to meet any government standards. However, "registration" is a limited and potentially misleading description of such a system, for it refers only to the role that government would play and ignores the private certification and reputation systems that would emerge in response to consumer demand.

Under a system of government registration, private organizations such as medical schools and medical specialty boards (and even the remnants of licensing boards) would develop standards and test physicians and other practitioners. These professional groups would grant their seal of approval to those they certify as competent to practice, and would advertise their "brand" to consumers. Competition for patients would drive providers to obtain certification.

Competition would keep both the certifying bodies and doctors focused on integrity and high-quality service. Boston College law professor Charles Baron explains:

> Under a voluntary system of private certification, the various certifying groups would have a direct financial and professional stake in acting intelligently and responsibly. Unlike state licensing boards, private certifying groups would face competition. If there were a number of different certifying groups, the value of each certificate would depend upon the standards of the group. Neither doctors nor patients would attach much importance to gaining certification from a group with lax, vague, or unsound standards.[73]

Practitioners would advertise their certifications to patients as well as their ratings from consumer groups such as in the *Consumers'*

Guide to Top Doctors. Consumer groups would not only rate providers, but rate the quality of certification boards as well.

A regime of government registration and private certification would also protect the public from incompetent practitioners. First, patients would police providers. As with laser eye surgery, patients would shop for experience and reputation rather than the cheapest provider. Second, while licensing boards currently do little to discipline inept providers, private certifying bodies would have to monitor the providers they certify and even revoke certifications in order to preserve their credibility. Finally, the courts would deter malpractice and compensate the injured.

FTC and IOM Recommendations

While encouraging further study of certification as an alternative to licensing, the FTC recommends that states "consider adopting the recommendation of the Institute of Medicine to broaden the membership of state licensure boards."[74] With many licensing boards dominated by the regulated profession, they have been able to restrict entry into the profession and the number of tasks that can be performed by those outside the profession. In contrast,

> State licensure boards with broader membership, including representatives of the general public, and individuals with expertise in health administration, economics, consumer affairs, education, and health services research, could be less likely to limit competition by [allied health professionals] and new business forms for the delivery of health care, and are less likely to engage in conduct that unreasonably increases prices or lowers access to health care.[75]

The FTC further urges states to adopt uniform licensing standards or reciprocity compacts that would give providers more freedom to practice telemedicine or relocate to another state. A better recommendation comes from the American Telemedicine Association, which encourages states not to regulate virtual medical consultations that take place across state borders.

These would be welcome changes that would restore the freedom of many providers and expand access for patients. Yet state governments should go farther. Liberalizing medical licensure would benefit patients and medical professionals. By increasing the supply of physicians and allied health professionals, as well as experimentation with new practice settings and modes of delivery, liberalization would increase competition, give patients a wider choice of providers, and lower the cost of medical care. By forcing providers to market themselves aggressively, greater competition would educate patients about medicine and the costs and benefits of different practitioners and types of practice.

Benefits would flow to providers as well. Allied health professionals and many physicians would have greater freedom to practice medicine how and where they choose. In particular, liberalizing licensure and scope-of-practice laws would give physician practices greater flexibility in assigning duties among their staff. Nonphysician clinicians, such as PAs and NPs, can lower costs and give physicians more time to focus on their comparative advantage.[76]

Barriers to Hospital Competition

States and the federal government have also erected barriers to the introduction of health care facilities. As discussed earlier, the federal moratorium on physician-owned specialty hospitals is one such barrier. State "certificate of need" (CON) laws are another. Currently, 35 states have such laws that require hospitals, nursing homes, and other facilities to obtain state approval before they may build a new facility, expand an existing facility, or offer new services. In such proceedings, it is common for competitors to have much to say about whether a new facility is needed. The FTC notes that numerous studies show "[m]arket incumbents can too easily use CON procedures to forestall competitors from entering an incumbent's market."[77]

The result is less competition, fewer choices for patients, higher prices, and reduced quality. According to the U.S. Government Accountability Office, 83 percent of specialty hospitals exist in states without CON laws, even though such states account for only 50 percent of the U.S. population and 55 percent of general hospitals.[78] Although CON laws were originally intended to control health care costs, studies have demonstrated they have had the opposite effect.[79] One study even found evidence that "mothers in states with certificate of need regulation are less likely to have a healthy baby."[80]

Like other barriers to competition, CON laws serve special interests at the expense of other providers and the public at large. The FTC advises, "States with Certificate of Need programs should reconsider whether these programs best serve their citizens' health care needs."[81] In fact, states should go further and repeal CON laws and other laws that block competition among providers.

Licensure is a long-neglected area of health policy, but one that deserves serious attention and significant reform. In 2005, President Bush proposed increasing federal spending on community health centers to $2 billion in fiscal year 2006 in an effort to establish "a health center in every high-poverty county that can support one."[82] Liberalizing state medical licensure laws, however, would enable more medical providers to experiment with low-cost ways of providing services to low-income areas without the need for additional tax dollars. A good way to do more for such Americans would be for government to do less.

8. Medical Malpractice Reform

Tort law is an important protection against those who do or would injure us, yet many complain—with some reason—that the medical liability "system" in the United States is out of control. Frivolous lawsuits are frequent, damages are exorbitant, and the aggrieved patients receive only a fraction of the monetary awards. Many specialists (neurosurgeons and obstetricians, to name two) report they cannot afford the rising cost of medical liability insurance, and have left states with high malpractice awards. Critics note that the fear of liability forces providers to practice "defensive medicine," including unnecessary but costly tests ordered merely to protect against potential liability. These and other costs of the medical tort system impose a significant burden on patients and taxpayers. Conover estimates the U.S. medical tort system provides benefits of $33.0 billion, but imposes costs of $113.7 billion, for a net cost of $80.7 billion per year.[1]

President George W. Bush has proposed federal legislation to limit medical malpractice awards. However, the U.S. Constitution does not grant Congress the authority to impose substantive rules of tort law on the states.[2] While the federal government may enact technical procedural changes, state legislatures are the proper venue for correcting excesses in state civil justice systems. The fact that medical professionals can avoid states with inhospitable civil justice systems gives them significant leverage when advocating state-level medical liability reforms, and gives states incentives to enact such reforms. That some states have done so further demonstrates that federal legislation is unnecessary. Michael Greve of the American Enterprise Institute notes, "At least so long as state law is trending in an anti-liability direction, experimentation is quite probably preferable to a federal 'reform' that might get it wrong, rob the reform states of their just rewards, and discourage laggard states from experimenting with their own, possibly more effective reforms."[3]

What reforms might states consider? Arbitrary caps on damages may reduce the costs of frivolous lawsuits, but they foreclose adequate relief in extreme cases, and prevent patients from bargaining for greater protection. A "loser pays" rule often would reallocate the costs of frivolous lawsuits to the correct party. However, it also would deter less affluent patients from seeking legal redress for legitimate grievances. One study found that "abolishing joint and several liability, restricting attorney's fees, and establishing victims' compensation funds all lead to fewer physicians per capita" within a state. Moreover, it is possible that arbitrary limits on liability will diminish incentives for marginal providers to exercise due care. The study also found that reducing awards to victims who also collect from insurance is associated with an increase in infant mortality.[4]

More patient-friendly and liberty-enhancing reforms would allow patients and providers to avoid the costly medical tort system via contract. Patients could choose the level of protection against malpractice they desire, rather than have that level imposed on them by the courts. Patients would select providers who offer acceptable levels of compensation for injuries caused by negligence. In cases of intentional wrongdoing or reckless behavior, tort rules would still apply. Providers could offer patients a menu of compensation options and their prices. Many providers likely would agree to high maximum awards to protect against the risk of an astronomical jury award. Supporters of legislative caps on damages could choose those limits for themselves. Patients who do not wish to limit their protections would be free to do that as well. Enforcing such contracts would mean that *patients*—not legislatures or the courts—would make tradeoffs between protecting themselves against immediate risks (the illness for which they seek treatment) and more remote risks (potential injuries from negligence).

One likely result would be more and better information on provider quality. Before agreeing to reduce their ability to recover damages, patients would demand information about providers' malpractice histories, something patients rarely do today. And numerous sources of information could help patients make their decisions. Consumer advocates (e.g., *Consumers' Guide to Top Doctors*) could evaluate different providers and the advantages and perils of different levels of malpractice protection. Competing providers would advertise the benefits of the protections they offer, including providers who refuse to limit their liability. Malpractice attorneys could advertise on television against the evils of negotiated limits on medical malpractice awards.

Another result would likely be greater innovation. As John Goodman and Gerald Musgrave suggest:

> [O]ne sensible way to cut down on the litigation costs for simple negligence would be to have the hospital take out a life insurance policy on a patient prior to surgery. The hospital and the patient (or the patient's family) could agree that if the patient dies for any reason, the beneficiaries will accept the policy's payment as full compensation, even if there was negligence. The same principle could apply to other injuries, such as disability leading to a loss of income. Litigation costs would be avoided, and life insurance companies would have incentives to monitor the quality of hospital care.[5]

On an individual basis and by mutual assent, patients and providers would reduce the costs of the tort system while improving the quality of medical care.

As Goodman and Musgrave note, "The current legal system ignores contractual waivers of tort liability. What is needed is a legal change requiring the courts to honor certain types of contracts under which tort claims are waived in return for compensation."[6]

Courts that refuse to enforce such contracts effectively require patients to purchase a level of malpractice protection that has been set by someone else. That restricts both patient freedom and access to health care, particularly for less affluent patients. George Mason University law professor Michael Krauss argues that the courts' failure to enforce contracts where patients agree to assume a greater risk effectively imposes a tax on poorer patients. "If unable to purchase anything but the highest quality, many poorer consumers will choose not to purchase at all," he writes. "They may even forgo medical treatment if tort law imposes Park Avenue pricing on the rural practitioner." "Today's torts 'crisis' does not exist because corporations are oppressing individuals, or because we need federal legislation to replace state tort rules. The crisis exists because our rights have been given increasingly less respect by government."[7]

Finally, American patients already have the freedom to choose their malpractice protections by traveling abroad for medical care. As discussed in the Introduction, Howard Staab found heart surgery was far less expensive in India than in North Carolina. That was in part due to different legal rules governing medical malpractice, as

145

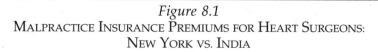

Figure 8.1
MALPRACTICE INSURANCE PREMIUMS FOR HEART SURGEONS:
NEW YORK VS. INDIA

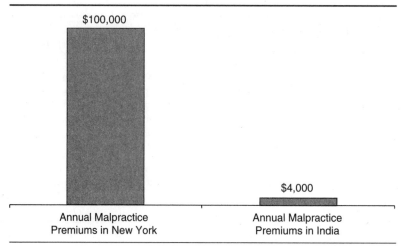

$100,000

$4,000

| Annual Malpractice | Annual Malpractice |
| Premiums in New York | Premiums in India |

SOURCE: John Lancaster, "Surgeries, Side Trips for 'Medical Tourists';
Affordable Care at India's Private Hospitals Draws Growing Number of
Foreigners," *Washington Post*, October 21, 2004, p. A1.

reflected in his surgeon's relatively low malpractice insurance premiums. Dr. Naresh Trehan noted that while a New York heart surgeon can pay $100,000 a year for malpractice insurance, Indian heart surgeons pay only $4,000 (see Figure 8.1).[8] It makes little sense to force Americans to leave the United States to exercise this freedom.

Some will object that patients need all the protections that U.S. courts can provide. Commenting on Staab's decision, a spokeswoman for the Centers for Disease Control cautioned, "If you travel outside this nation, the same protections that are built into the healthcare delivery system here may not apply."[9] But that is precisely the point: some patients cannot afford those protections. To save his life, Howard Staab had to negotiate around the malpractice protections and other aspects of the U.S. health care system that put heart surgery out of reach.

Restricting patients' freedom to make such decisions for themselves makes them less safe. Patients would be better served by a competitive process that acknowledges that one size does not fit all, allows patients to choose among diverse approaches to malpractice protection, and rejects those that do not work. If the courts will not respect Americans' right to make such contracts here at home, legislators should ensure that such contracts will be enforced.

Conclusion

Despite its marvels, America's health care sector continues to present troubling symptoms: excessive costs, uneven quality, a lack of useful information for patients and providers, extraordinary waste, and enormous burdens for future taxpayers. An accurate diagnosis points to too much government influence and too little choice and competition. Proposals to increase the role of government would aggravate these symptoms. More subsidies or controls would drain from the medical marketplace even more of the dynamics that drive *other* sectors of the economy toward lower prices and higher quality. The only sure remedy is to restore those dynamics to the health care sector.

Although there are dark clouds on the horizon, we are heartened by the creation and steady growth of health savings accounts. HSAs have already begun to change private-sector health care from within, and will enable a reexamination of the role of government in health care. It is one thing to impose costly regulations on consumers—such as requiring them to purchase coverage for acupuncture and hairpieces—when it seems that employers are paying the bill. It will be more difficult to do so when the cost is apparent to millions of individual consumers.

HSAs also represent a down payment on reform of government health programs.[1] First, they will help to contain medical inflation by making millions of consumers more price-sensitive. That will benefit all payers, including taxpayers. Second, experience with HSAs will accustom Americans to exercising more control over their own health care. That may make Americans more comfortable with experimenting with HSAs in government health programs. In particular, as more HSA holders reach age 65, they could form a powerful constituency for Medicare reforms based on choice and competition. It is one thing for the federal government to make health care decisions for retirees when those retirees are already accustomed to surrendering control over such decisions to their employers. It will become more difficult for government to do so if workers are accustomed to making their own health care and insurance decisions. Finally, HSAs enable today's workers to save for their retirement health expenses and can help build support for prefunding Medicare through personal savings accounts.

We are heartened by the creation of health savings accounts for more than these reasons, though. HSAs represent a moral victory for freedom and competition in health care. We are eager to see how health care will change as health savings accounts restore to patients and providers much of the autonomy that has been eroded by decades of increasing government control.

However, HSAs alone will not fully restore choice and competition to America's health care sector. That will require returning control over the nation's health care dollars to the workers who earned them. State and federal lawmakers should build on the success of HSAs by applying these principles to all areas of health policy: tax reform, government health programs, the medical tort system, and regulation of health insurance, pharmaceuticals, medical devices, providers, and the allocation of transplantable organs. In particular, Congress should use HSAs as a model for prefunding Medicare's enormous future obligations through personal savings accounts.

The competitive market process will do a better job than government of making medical care of ever-increasing quality available to an ever-increasing number of consumers. We have seen competition deliver higher quality and lower prices in other areas of the economy. As Michael Porter and Elizabeth Teisberg write:

> It is often argued that health care is different because it is complex; because consumers have limited information; and because services are highly customized. Health care undoubtedly has these characteristics, but so do other industries where competition works well. For example, the business of providing customized software and technical services to corporations is highly complex, yet, when adjusted for quality, the cost of enterprise computing has fallen dramatically over the last decade.[2]

Although we share Porter and Teisberg's view, we also share one view held by many proponents of government activism in the health care sector: health care is a special area of the economy. Unlike software, wireless communications, or banking, health care involves very emotional decisions, which often entail matters of human dignity, life, and death. However, we do not see the gravity of these matters as a reason to divert power away from individuals and toward government. Rather, we see the special nature of health care as all the more reason to increase each consumer's sphere of autonomy. The special nature of health care makes it all the more important that we use the competitive process to make health care available to more consumers—and makes it all the more important to get started now.

Notes

Preface

1. Beth Fouhy, "Clinton Outlines Legislative Priorities," Associated Press, November 13, 2006.

2. Scott Helman, "Mass Bill Requires Health Insurance," *Boston Globe*, April 4, 2006. For a detailed critique of the Massachusetts plan, see Michael Tanner, "No Miracle in Massachusetts: Why Governor Romney's Health Care Reform Won't Work," Cato Institute Briefing Paper no. 97, June 6, 2006.

3. Jennifer Steinhauer, "California Plan for Health Care Would Cover All," *New York Times*, January 9, 2007.

4. Michael F. Cannon, "Schwarzenegger's Health-Care Shakedown," *National Review Online*, January 22, 2007, http://article.nationalreview.com/?q = ZWJiZTBjYm FjYzdkODc4YmVmMDUzNzliZTA5YThlOGM = .

5. Dan Balz, "At Forum, Democrats Differ on Health Care; Funding Plans Include Raising Taxes, Ending War, Reshaping the Insurance System," *Washington Post*, March 25, 2007, p. A05.

Introduction

1. F. A. Hayek, "Competition as a Discovery Procedure," *The Quarterly Journal of Austrian Economics* 5, no. 3 (Fall 2002), p. 9, http://www.mises.org/journals/qjae/pdf/qjae5_3_3.pdf.

2. F. A. Hayek, *Law, Legislation and Liberty, vol. 3: The Political Order of a Free People* (Chicago: University of Chicago Press, 1979), p. 68.

3. Hayek, see note 1, pp. 9–23.

4. Michael E. Porter and Elizabeth Teisberg, "Redefining Competition in Health Care," *Harvard Business Review*, online edition, June 1, 2004.

5. Ibid.

6. The exception is generic prices in Canada, which are "6 percent lower than U.S. generic prices." Patricia M. Danzon and Michael F. Furukawa, "Prices and Availability of Pharmaceuticals: Evidence from Nine Countries," *Health Affairs* Web Exclusive, October 29, 2003, pp. W3-528, 534, http://content.healthaffairs.org/cgi/reprint/hlthaff.w3.521v1.pdf.

7. Kenneth I. Kaitin, ed., "Incremental R&D Creates Safer, More Effective Drugs & Fosters Competition," *Tufts Center for the Study of Drug Development* Impact Report no. 6, November/December 2004, p. 6; release available at http://csdd.tufts.edu./NewsEvents/RecentNews.asp?newsid = 48.

8. John C. Goodman, "Health Care in a Free Society: Rebutting the Myths of National Health Insurance," Cato Institute Policy Analysis no. 532, p. 16, http://www.cato.org/pubs/pas/pa532.pdf.

9. David Harmon, *Comprehensive Report on the Refractive Market* (Manchester, Mo.: Market Scope, October 2004), p. 62, see http://www.mktsc.com/refractive%20report. html.

10. See Sean O'Neill, "Eyes on the Price," *Kiplinger's Personal Finance Magazine* 54, no. 9, September 2000, p. 122; and Karen Garloch (*The Charlotte Observer*), "Vision Quest; Laser eye surgery is popular, despite slight risks," *Monterey County Herald*, March 14, 2004.

11. Lisette Hilton, "Keep the Faith; Experts predict that laser vision correction's recovery comes on the heels of economic upturn," *Review of Refractive Surgery* 3, no. 1, February 15, 2002, http://www.reviewofrefractivesurgery.com/index.asp?page=6_1.htm.

12. Jay Solomon, "India's New Coup in Outsourcing: Inpatient Care," *Wall Street Journal*, April 26, 2004, p. A1.

13. Saritha Rai, "Low Costs Lure Foreigners to India for Medical Care," *New York Times*, April 7, 2005, p. C6, http://www.nytimes.com/2005/04/07/business/worldbusiness/07health.html.

14. Kadi Hodges, "Man in India for Heart Surgery," *Herald-Sun* (Durham), September 27, 2004, http://www.heraldsun.com/tools/printfriendly.cfm?StoryID=526723; and Vicki Cheng, "Americans increasingly find health care abroad," *News & Observer* (Raleigh), September 23, 2004, http://www.newsobserver.com/news/nc/v-printer/story/1664206p-7897201c.html.

15. John Lancaster, "Surgeries, Side Trips for 'Medical Tourists'; Affordable Care at India's Private Hospitals Draws Growing Number of Foreigners," *Washington Post*, October 21, 2004, p. A1, http://www.washingtonpost.com/wp-dyn/articles/A49743-2004Oct20.html.

16. Solomon, see note 12.

17. Rai, see note 13.

18. Ibid.

19. Lancaster, see note 15.

20. Rai, see note 13; and Solomon, see note 12.

21. Rai, see note 13.

22. Lancaster, see note 15.

23. Ibid.

24. Ibid.

25. Solomon, see note 12.

26. Daniel P. Kessler and Mark B. McClellan, "Is Hospital Competition Socially Wasteful?" NBER Working Paper no. w7266, July 1999, pp. 28–29, 37, http://dsl.nber.org/papers/w7266.pdf.

27. Daniel P. Kessler and Jeffrey J. Geppert, "The Effects of Competition on Variation in the Quality and Cost of Medical Care," NBER Working Paper no. 11226, March 2005, p. 2, http://papers.nber.org/tmp/10007-w11226.pdf.

28. U.S. Federal Trade Commission/Department of Justice, *Improving Health Care: A Dose of Competition*, July 23, 2004, Executive Summary, p. 20, http://www.ftc.gov/reports/healthcare/040723healthcarerpt.pdf.

29. Alain Enthoven, "The History and Principles of Managed Competition," *Health Affairs*, Supplement (1993): 44, http://emlab.berkeley.edu/users/webfac/held/157_VC2.pdf.

30. George Silver, "Health Care: Beyond Markets," *Washington Post*, November 11, 2004, p. A37, http://www.washingtonpost.com/wp-dyn/articles/A41307-2004Nov10.html.

31. Patricia M. Danzon, "Health Care Industry," *The Concise Encyclopedia of Economics*, 1993, http://www.econlib.org/library/Enc/HealthCareIndustry.html.

32. U.S. Bureau of Labor Statistics/Bureau of the Census, "Table HI01. Health Insurance Coverage Status and Type of Coverage by Selected Characteristics: 2003," http://ferret.bls.census.gov/macro/032004/health/h01_001.htm.

33. U.S. Federal Trade Commission, "Joint FTC/Department of Justice Hearing on Health Care and Competition Law and Policy," transcript, May 29, 2003, p. 148, http://www.ftc.gov/ogc/healthcarehearings/030529ftctrans.pdf.

Chapter 1

1. "Nobel Prize in Physiology or Medicine Winners 2004–1901[sic]," The Nobel Prize Internet Archive, accessed December 1, 2004, http://almaz.com/nobel/medicine/medicine.html.

2. Pharmaceutical Manufacturers Association, "Facts about the U.S. Pharmaceutical Industry," 2002, http://www.phrma.org/publications/publications/brochure/leading/lead9.cfm.

3. *Economic Report of the President* (Washington: U.S. Government Printing Office, February 2004), p. 192, http://www.gpoaccess.gov/eop/.

4. Gerard F. Anderson, Uwe E. Reinhardt, Peter S. Hussey, and Varduhi Petrosyan, "It's the Prices, Stupid: Why the United States Is So Different from Other Countries," *Health Affairs* 22, no. 3, Exhibit 5 (May/June 2003): 99, http://content.healthaffairs.org/cgi/reprint/22/3/89.pdf; and Stephen Pollard, "European Health Care Consensus Group Paper," Centre for the New Europe, January 4, 2001, as cited in John Goodman, Gerald Musgrave, and Devon Herrick, *Lives at Risk: Single-Payer National Health Care around the World* (New York: Rowman and Littlefield, 2004). A variation of Figure 1.1 originally appeared in Goodman et al., p. 63.

5. Data on breast cancer, colon cancer, lung cancer, and heart attacks come from Gerard F. Anderson, Varduhi Petrosyan, and Peter S. Hussey, "Multinational Comparisons of Health Systems Data, 2002," Commonwealth Fund, October 2002, pp. 55–62. Data on prostate cancer and AIDS come from Gerard F. Anderson and Peter S. Hussey, "Multinational Comparisons of Health Systems Data," Commonwealth Fund, October 2000, pp. 17–18. The studies use OECD data, which the authors describe thus: "Working with statistical offices in each member country, the OECD produces the most accurate and comprehensive international health care data available on the 30 nations. . . . Although every effort was made to standardize the comparisons, countries inevitably differ in their definitions of terms. Furthermore, some of the numbers are preliminary estimates. Wherever possible, the most recent year with relatively complete data was used; however, data from earlier years was sometimes substituted when the most recent data were not available for a specific country. The comparisons should therefore be seen as guides to relative orders of magnitude rather than as indicators of precise differences" (2002, p. 1).

6. Steve Findlay, "U.S. Hospitals Attracting Patients from Abroad," *USA Today*, July 22, 1997.

7. Robert Blendon et al., "Physicians' Perspectives on Caring for Patients in the United States, Canada, and West Germany," *The New England Journal of Medicine* 328, no. 14 (April 8, 1993): 1011–1016.

8. John C. Goodman, "Health Care in a Free Society: Rebutting the Myths of National Health Insurance," Cato Institute Policy Analysis no. 532, p. 7, http://www.cato.org/pubs/pas/pa532.pdf.

9. Centers for Medicare & Medicaid Services, Office of the Actuary, "Table 1: National Health Expenditures and Selected Economic Indicators, Levels and Annual Percent Change: Calendar Years 2001–2016," http://www.cms.hhs.gov/ NationalHealthExpendData/downloads/proj2006.pdf.

10. Organization for Economic Cooperation and Development, *OECD Health Data 2006*, October 10, 2006, "Total Expenditure on Health, %GDP," http://www.oecd.org/ dataoecd/20/51/37622205.xls, authors' calculations.

11. Centers for Medicare & Medicaid Services, see note 9.

12. *Budget of the United States Government, Fiscal Year 2008* (Washington: Government Printing Office, February 2007), p. 43, http://www.gpoaccess.gov/usbudget/ fy08/browse.html; and "Table 57. Age of reference person: Shares of annual aggregate expenditures and sources of income," U.S. Department of Labor, Bureau of Labor Statistics, Consumer Expenditures Survey, 2005, http://www.bls.gov/cex/2005/ Aggregate/age.pdf.

13. Uwe E. Reinhardt, Peter S. Hussey, and Gerard F. Anderson, "U.S. Health Care Spending in an International Context," *Health Affairs* 23, no. 3 (May/June 2004): 11–12, http://content.healthaffairs.org/cgi/reprint/23/3/10.pdf.

14. Charles I. Jones, "Why Have Health Expenditures As a Share of GDP Risen So Much?" Version 3.0, May 5, 2004, p. 8, http://elsa.berkeley.edu/~chad/health 300.pdf.

15. Frank R. Lichtenberg, "The Effect of Pharmaceutical Utilization and Innovation on Hospitalization and Mortality," NBER Working Paper no. 5418, January 1996, http://www.nber.org/papers/W5418.

16. Frank R. Lichtenberg, "Sources of U.S. Longevity Increase, 1960–1997," NBER Working Paper no. 8755, February 2002, p. 11, http://www.nber.org/papers/W8755.

17. Mark G. Duggan and William N. Evans, "Estimating the Impact of Medical Innovation: The Case of HIV Antiretroviral Treatments," NBER Working Paper no. 11109, February 2005, p. 1, http://www.nber.org/papers/w11109.

18. Ibid., American Heart Association, *Heart Disease and Stroke Statistics—2005 Update*, p. 51.

19. Frank R. Lichtenberg, "The Impact of New Drug Launches on Longevity: Evidence from Longitudinal, Disease-Level Data from 52 Countries, 1982–2001," NBER Working Paper no. 9754, June 2003, p. 21, http://www.nber.org/papers/ w9754.

20. Jones, see note 14.

21. David M. Cutler and Mark McClellan, "Is Technological Change in Medicine Worth It?" *Health Affairs* 20, no. 5 (September/October 2001): 11–29, http://content. healthaffairs.org/cgi/reprint/20/5/11.pdf.

22. David M. Cutler, Mark B. McClellan, Joseph P. Newhouse, and Dahlia Remler, "Are Medical Prices Declining? Evidence from Heart Attack Treatments," *Quarterly Journal of Economics* 113, no. 4 (November 1998): 991–1024.

23. Irving Shapiro, Matthew D. Shapiro, and David W. Wilcox, "Measuring the Value of Cataract Surgery," University of Michigan mimeo, 1999; cited in Jones, see note 14.

24. Ernst R. Berndt, Anupa Bir, Susan H. Busch, Richard G. Frank, and Shaon-Lise T. Normand, "The Medical Treatment of Depression, 1991–1996: Productive Inefficiency, Expected Outcome Variations, and Price Indexes," NBER Working Paper no. 7816, July 2000, http://www.nber.org/papers/W7816.

25. Steve Lohr, "Health Care Costs Are a Killer, But Maybe That's a Plus," *New York Times*, September 26, 2004.

26. *Economic Report of the President* (Washington: U.S. Government Printing Office, February 2004), p. 191, http://www.gpoaccess.gov/eop/.

27. Organization for Economic Cooperation and Development, "Infant mortality, deaths per 1,000 live births," *OECD Health Data 2004*, 3rd ed., http://www.oecd.org/dataoecd/13/40/31963124.xls.

28. Miranda Mugford, "A Comparison of Reported Differences in Definitions of Vital Events and Statistics," *World Health Statistics Quarterly* 36 (1983): 205; quoted in Nicholas Eberstadt, *The Tyranny of Numbers: Measurement & Misrule* (Washington: AEI Press, 1995), p. 50.

29. Eberstadt, p. 54.

30. Organization for Economic Cooperation and Development, "OECD Health Data 2004—Frequently Requested Data," June 3, 2004, tables 1–2, 9–10, http://www.oecd.org/document/16/0,2340,en_2649_37407_2085200_1_1_1_37407,00.html. All data are for 2002, except life expectancy data for South Korea, the United Kingdom and the United States (2001); per capita health expenditures for Japan (2001); and GDP data for Turkey (2000).

Chapter 2

1. "NABE Panel to Next President: Concentrate on Terror, not Stimulus," *National Association for Business Economics Economic Policy Survey*, August 17, 2004, p. 1, http://www.nabe.com/publib/pol/04/pol0408.pdf.

2. Ruth Helman and Paul Fronstin, "Public Attitudes on the U.S. Health Care System: Findings from the Health Confidence Survey," EBRI *Issue Brief* no. 275, November 2004, p. 7, http://www.ebri.org/EBRI.HCS04.pdf.

3. Sara R. Collins, Cathy Schoen, Michelle M. Doty, and Alyssa L. Holmgren, "Job-Based Health Insurance in the Balance: Employer Views of Coverage in the Workplace," The Commonwealth Fund Issue Brief, no. 718, March 2004, p. 7, http://www.cmwf.org/usr_doc/collins_jobbased_718.pdf.

4. U.S. Congressional Budget Office, *The Budget and Economic Outlook: Fiscal Years 2008 to 2017*, January 2007, p. 50, 54, http://www.cbo.gov/ftpdocs/77xx/doc7731/01-24-BudgetOutlook.pdf.

5. Ibid., p. 50.

6. U.S. Congressional Budget Office, *The Long-Term Budget Outlook, 2005*, December 2005, p. 22, http://www.cbo.gov/ftpdocs/69xx/doc6982/12-15-LongTermOutlook.pdf.

7. Author's calculations, from *2007 Annual Report of the Board of Trustees of the Federal Hospital Insurance and Federal Supplementary Medical Insurance Trust Funds* (Washington: Government Printing Office, April 23, 2007), pp. 67, 105, 120, http://www.cms.hhs.gov/ReportsTrustFunds/downloads/tr2007.pdf.

8. Elizabeth A. McGlynn et al., "The Quality of Health Care Delivered to Adults in the United States," *New England Journal of Medicine* 348 (June 26, 2003): 2635–45.

9. Institute of Medicine, *Crossing the Quality Chasm: A New Health System for the 21st Century* (Washington: National Academy Press, 2001).

10. HealthGrades, Inc., "Patient Safety in American Hospitals," July 2004, pp. 5–6, http://www.healthgrades.com/media/english/pdf/HG_Patient_Safety_Study_Final.pdf.

11. Christopher P. Landrigan et al., "Effect of Reducing Interns' Work Hours on Serious Medical Errors in Intensive Care Units," *New England Journal of Medicine* 351,

no. 18 (October 28, 2004): 1838–48; and Steven W. Lockley et al., "Effect of Reducing Interns' Weekly Work Hours on Sleep and Attentional Failures," *New England Journal of Medicine* 351, no. 18 (October 28, 2004): 1829–37.

12. David P. Phillips, Jason R. Jarvinen, and Rosalie R. Phillips, "A Spike in Fatal Medication Errors at the Beginning of Each Month," *Pharmacotherapy* 25, no. 1 (January 2005): 1–9.

13. Barbara Starfield, "Is U.S. Health Really the Best in the World?" *Journal of the American Medical Association* 284, no. 4 (July 26, 2000): 483.

14. *Health Care in Canada 2004* (Ottawa: Canadian Institute for Health Information, 2004), p. 42, http://secure.cihi.ca/cihiweb/products/hcic2004_e.pdf. The population of the United States is roughly nine times that of Canada. "Population in 1999 and 2000: All Countries," United Nations, Population Division, Department of Economic and Social Affairs, p. 5, http://www.un.org/popin/popdiv/pop1999-00.pdf.

15. In surveys, 24 percent of Canadians reported that they or a family member had experienced a "preventable adverse event" *in the past year* [*Health Care in Canada 2004* (Ottawa: Canadian Institute for Health Information, 2004), p. 43, http://secure.cihi.ca/cihiweb/products/hcic2004_e.pdf], compared with 34 percent of Americans who reported they or a family member had *ever* experienced a "preventable medical error" ("National Survey on Consumers' Experiences with Patient Safety and Quality Information," Kaiser Family Foundation, November 2004, p. 17, http://www.kff.org/kaiserpolls/loader.cfm?url=/commonspot/security/getfile.cfm&PageID=48814).

16. Laura Eggertson, "Quebec Strikes Committee on *Clostridium Difficile*," *Canadian Medical Association Journal* 171, no. 2 (July 20, 2004): 123, http://www.cmaj.ca/cgi/reprint/171/2/123.pdf.

17. "Summary Report: 2004 Survey of Physicians 50 to 65 Years Old," Merritt, Hawkins & Associates, http://www.merritthawkins.com/pdf/2004_physician50_survey.pdf.

18. Bruce E. Landon, James Reschovsky, and David Blumenthal, "Changes in Career Satisfaction among Primary Care and Specialist Physicians, 1997–2001," *Journal of the American Medical Association* 289, no. 4 (January 22, 2003): 442–449.

Chapter 3

1. "One Single Solution: Doctors Call for Single-Payer Health Care," *Dissident Voice*, August 18, 2003.

2. Alice Dembner, "Kennedy to Propose Universal Health Care," *Boston Globe*, January 22, 2004.

3. Alan J. Borsuk, "Kerry Vows to Fight for Health Care," *Milwaukee Journal-Sentinel*, September 14, 2004.

4. For one such proposal, see H.J.Res. 30 (108th Congress), introduced by Rep. Jesse L. Jackson Jr., March 4, 2003.

5. J. D. Kleinke, "Access versus Excess: Value-Based Cost Sharing for Prescription Drugs," *Health Affairs* 23, no. 1 (2004): 34–47, http://content.healthaffairs.org/cgi/reprint/23/1/34.

6. One possible delineation would be between emergency and nonemergency care. However, federal law already requires emergency rooms to screen and stabilize all patients regardless of ability to pay. Thus, effectively, Americans already enjoy a legislatively mandated "right" to emergency care.

7. Jim O'Sullivan and Priscilla Yeon, "Lawmakers Nix Petition Guaranteeing Health Care Access," *State House News Service*, January 2, 2007, http://www. healthcareformass.org/press/documents/LAWMAKERSNIXPETITION GUARANTEEINGHEALTHCAREACCESS.pdf.

8. John C. Goodman, "Health Care in a Free Society: Rebutting the Myths of National Health Insurance," Cato Institute Policy Analysis no. 532, p. 3, http:// www.cato.org/pubs/pas/pa532.pdf.

9. Ibid., p. 20.

10. John Goodman, Gerald Musgrave, and Devon Herrick, *Lives at Risk: Single-Payer National Health Care around the World* (New York: Rowman and Littlefield, 2004), p. vii.

11. "Health Care Reform a Major Theme in Presidential Race," *The Commonwealth Fund Quarterly* 9, no. 3 (Fall 2003): 4.

12. Patricia M. Danzon, "Hidden Overhead Costs: Is Canada's System Really Less Expensive?" *Health Affairs* 11, no. 1 (Spring 1992): 21–43, http://content.healthaffairs. org/cgi/reprint/11/1/21.pdf.

13. Valerie Elliott, " 'Bed Blockers' Farmed Out for B&B Recovery," *The Times* (London), February 9, 2002; "Statistical Press Notice: NHS Waiting List Figures—28 February 2002," U.K. Department of Health, April 5, 2002.

14. "Purchasing for Your Health 1996/97," New Zealand Ministry of Health, March 1998, cited in Goodman et al., see note 10, p. 18.

15. Wess Mitchell, "Sweden Edges toward Free-Market Medicine," NCPA Brief Analysis no. 369, August 31, 2001, http://www.ncpa.org/pub/ba/ba369.

16. Cathy Schoen et al., "Comparison of Health Care System Views and Experiences in Five Nations, 2001," Commonwealth Fund Issue Brief, no. 542, May 2002, p. 4, http://www.cmwf.org/usr_doc/Schoen _5nationcomparison_542.pdf.

17. Nadeem Esmail and Michael A. Walker, "Waiting Your Turn: Hospital Waiting Lists in Canada, 14th Edition," Fraser Institute, *Critical Issues Bulletin*, October 2004.

18. David Green and Laura Casper, *Delay, Denial and Dilution: The Impact of NHS Rationing on Heart Disease and Cancer* (London: Institute of Economic Affairs, 2000).

19. "Canadian Health Care—A System in Collapse," Fraser Institute, *Backgrounder*, 1999.

20. David Harriman, William McArthur, and Martin Zelder, "The Availability of Medical Technology in Canada: An International Comparative Study," Fraser Institute, Public Policy Sources no. 28, August 6, 1999.

21. Gerard F. Anderson, Uwe E. Reinhardt, Peter S. Hussey, and Varduhi Petrosyan, "It's the Prices, Stupid: Why the United States Is So Different from Other Countries," *Health Affairs* 22, no. 3 (May/June 2003): 89–105.

22. Harriman et al., see note 20.

23. Anderson et al., see note 21.

24. Harriman et al., see note 20.

25. David Gratzer, *Code Blue: Reviving Canada's Health Care System* (Toronto: ECW Press, 1999), pp. 93–97.

26. "In 2003, the average Canadian family earned an income of $58,782 and paid total taxes equaling $27,640 (47.0 percent)." Figures are in Canadian dollars. "Tax Bill for the Average Canadian Family Has Increased 1550 Percent Since 1961," Fraser Institute news release, February 4, 2004, http://www.fraserinstitute.ca/shared/ readmore.asp?sNav = nr&id = 584.

27. American Medical Student Association, "Theoretical Models for Delivering Health Care," http://www.amsa.org/hp/theories.cfm.

28. Alain Enthoven, "The History and Principles of Managed Competition," *Health Affairs*, Supplement (1993): 44, http://emlab.berkeley.edu/users/webfac/held/157_VC2.pdf.

29. Chapter 58 of the Acts of 2006, section 101. The law defines the Connector as "a body politic and corporate and a public instrumentality." It is designed to operate independent of any other government agency and has a corporate charter, but its board consists of the Massachusetts secretary of administration and finance, the state Medicaid director, the state commissioner of insurance, the executive director of the group insurance commission, three members appointed by the governor, and three members appointed by the attorney general. As an entity it falls somewhere between a government agency and a private corporation. One useful analogy would be the Federal Reserve Board.

30. Robert Moffit and Nina Owcharenko, "Understanding Key Parts of the Massachusetts Health Plan," *Human Events Online*, April 21, 2006, http://www.humanevents.com/article.php?id = 14200.

31. Chapter 58 of the Massachusetts Acts of 2006, sections 101 and 76.

32. Richard Epstein, "Unmanageable Care," *Reason*, May 1993.

33. Enthoven, see note 28, p. 44.

34. Andrew Dick, "Will Employer Mandates Really Work? Another Look at Hawaii," *Health Affairs Update* [Spring (I) 1994]: 343–49, http://content.healthaffairs.org/cgi/reprint/13/1/343.pdf.

35. Smaller firms would have been required to finance coverage only for employees.

36. Anna D. Sinaiko, "Employers' Responses to a Play-or-Pay Mandate: An Analysis of California's Health Insurance Act of 2003," *Health Affairs Web Exclusive* (October 13, 2004): W4-469–79, http://content.healthaffairs.org/cgi/reprint/hlthaff.w4.469v1.pdf.

37. Aaron Yelowitz, "The Economic Impact of Proposition 72 on California Employers," Employment Policies Institute, September 2004, p. vi, http://www.epionline.org/studies/yelowitz_09-2004.pdf.

38. Dick, see note 34.

39. Sinaiko, see note 36.

40. Sara R. Collins, Cathy Schoen, Michelle M. Doty, and Alyssa L. Holmgren, "Job-Based Health Insurance in the Balance: Employer Views of Coverage in the Workplace," The Commonwealth Fund Issue Brief, no. 718, March 2004, p. 5, http://www.cmwf.org/usr_doc/collins_jobbased_718.pdf.

41. John Wagner and Michael Barbaro, "Md. Passes Rules on Wal-Mart Insurance," *Washington Post*, April 6, 2005.

42. Matthew Mosk and Ylan Mui, "Wal-Mart Law in Md. Rejected by Court," *Washington Post*, July 20, 2006.

43. Jennifer Steinhauer, "California Plan for Health Care Would Cover All," *New York Times*, January 9, 2007.

44. Claudia L. Schur, Marc L. Berk, and Jill M. Yegian, "Workers' Perspectives on Mandated Employer Health Insurance," *Health Affairs Web Exclusive*, March 17, 2004, p. W4-133, http://content.healthaffairs.org/cgi/reprint/hlthaff.w4.128v1.pdf.

45. See Michael Tanner, "Individual Mandates for Health Insurance: Slippery Slope to National Health Care," Cato Institute Policy Analysis no. 565, April 5, 2006.

46. Robert Hartman and Paul van de Water, "The Budgetary Treatment of an Individual Mandate to Buy Health Insurance," Congressional Budget Office Memorandum, August 1994.

47. Scott Helman, "Mass Bill Requires Health Insurance," *Boston Globe*, April 4, 2006. For a detailed critique of the Massachusetts plan, see Michael Tanner, "No Miracle in Massachusetts: Why Governor Romney's Health Care Reform Won't Work," Cato Institute Briefing Paper no. 97, June 6, 2006.

48. Insurance Research Council, "IRC Estimates More Than 14 Percent of Drivers Are Uninsured," news release, June 28, 2006, http://www.ircweb.org/news/20060628.pdf.

49. Stephanie Jones, "Uninsured Drivers Travel under the Radar," *Insurance Journal*, August 18, 2003.

50. Greg Kelly, "Can Government Force People to Buy Insurance?" *Council for Affordable Health Insurance's Issues & Answers*, no. 123 (March 2004).

51. Ibid.

52. Peter Orszag and Matthew Hall, "Non-filers and Filers with Modest Tax Liabilities," *Tax Notes*, Tax Policy Center, Urban Institute and Brookings Institution, August 4, 2003, http://www.urban.org/UploadedPDF/1000548_TaxFacts_080403.pdf.

53. Nina Olson, *National Taxpayer Advocate 2003 Annual Report to Congress*, Taxpayer Advocate Service, Internal Revenue Service, December 31, 2003, http://www.irs.gov/pub/irs-utl/nta_2003_annual_update_mcw_1-15-042.pdf.

54. C. Eugene Steuerle, "Implementing Employer and Individual Mandates," *Health Affairs* II (Spring 1994): 54.

55. Ibid., p. 62.

56. Massachusetts has some 40 mandated benefits, including treatment for alcoholism, blood lead poisoning, bone marrow transplants, breast reconstruction, cervical cancer/human papillomavirus screening, clinical trials, contraceptives, diabetic supplies, emergency services, hair prostheses, home health care, in vitro fertilization, mammograms, mastectomy, maternity care and maternity stays, mental health generally (in addition there is a requirement for mental health parity), newborn hearing screening, off-label drug use, phenylketonuria/formula, prostate screening, rehabilitation services, and well-child care. Services of the following providers must also be covered: chiropractors, dentists, nurse anesthetists, nurse midwives, optometrists, podiatrists, professional counselors, psychiatric nurses, psychologists, social workers, and speech or hearing therapists. Insurance policies must provide coverage to adopted children, handicapped dependents, and newborns. Victoria Craig Bunce, J. P. Wieske, and Vlasta Prikazky, "Health Insurance Mandates in the States, 2006," Council for Affordable Health Insurance, March 2006, http://www.aba.com/NR/rdonlyres/7DEC4FCA-57A0-4CC5-834A-22C9AB859D37/43015/CAHIState Mandates32006.pdf.

57. Quoted in Julie Appleby, "Mass. Gov. Romney's Health Care Plan Says Everyone Pays," *USA Today*, July 4, 2005.

58. Alice Dembner, "Health Plan May Exempt 20% of the Uninsured," *Boston Globe*, April 12, 2007; Julie Appleby, "Mass. Health Plan Finds Cost Is Too High for 20% of People," *USA Today*, April 13, 2007.

59. U.S. Centers for Medicare & Medicaid Services, "National Health Expenditure Projections 2006–2016," p. 6, http://www.cms.hhs.gov/NationalHealthExpendData/downloads/proj2006.pdf.

60. Kaiser Family Foundation/Health Research Educational Trust, *Employer Health Benefits 2006 Annual Survey*, p. 25, http://www.kff.org/insurance/7527/index.cfm.

Chapter 4

1. Authors' calculations from "Table 9: Total expenditure on health, Per capita US$ PPP," and "Table 16: Out-of-pocket payments, Per capita US$ PPP," *OECD Health Data 2004—Frequently Requested Data*, June 3, 2004, authors' files.

2. Sidney T. Bogardus Jr., David E. Geist, and Elizabeth H. Bradley, "Physicians' Interactions with Third-Party Payers: Is Deception Necessary?" *Archives of Internal Medicine* 164 (September 27, 2004): 1841–44, http://archinte.ama-assn.org/cgi/gca? gca = 164%2F17%2F1841&submit.x = 144&submit.y = 10.

3. Ibid.

4. Ibid.

5. Clifford J. Levy and Michael Luo, "New York Medicaid Fraud May Reach Into Billions," *New York Times*, July 18, 2005, p. A1.

6. U.S. General Accounting Office, "High-Risk Series: Medicare," GAO/HR-97-10, February 1997, p. 7.

7. Centers for Medicare & Medicaid Services, Office of the Actuary, "Table 1: National Health Expenditures and Selected Economic Indicators, Levels and Annual Percent Change: Calendar Years 2001–2016," http://www.cms.hhs.gov/NationalHealthExpendData/downloads/proj2006.pdf.

8. Center for Responsive Politics, "Industry Totals: Health," http://www.opensecrets.org/industries/indus.asp?Ind = H, and "Lobbyist Database," http://www.opensecrets.org/lobbyists/indus.asp?Ind = H; and Follow the Money, customized search, http://followthemoney.org/. According to the Center for Responsive Politics, "All numbers attributed to a particular industry can be assumed to be conservative," http://www.opensecrets.org/industries/methodology.asp. Lobbying expenditures may also be underestimated: "Spending by corporations, industry groups, unions and other interests that is not strictly for lobbying of government officials, but is still meant to influence public policy, is not reported—and may exceed what was spent on direct lobbying. Such activities include public relations, advertising and grassroots lobbying," http://www.opensecrets.org/pressreleases/2007/2006Lobbying.3.15.asp.

9. Center for Responsive Politics, "Lobbyist Spending by Sector in 2006," http://www.opensecrets.org/lobbyists/index.asp?showyear = 2006&txtindextype = c.

10. Center for Responsive Politics, "2006 Election Overview: Top Industries," http://www.opensecrets.org/overview/industries.asp?cycle = 2006. See also Center for Responsive Politics, "2006 Election Overview: Totals by Sector," http://www.opensecrets.org/overview/sectors.asp?Cycle = 2006&Bkdn = DemRep&Sortby = Rank.

11. Paul B. Ginsburg and Len M. Nichols, "The Health Care Cost-Coverage Conundrum: The Care We Want vs. the Care We Can Afford," Center for Studying Health System Change Commentary, Fall 2003, http://www.hschange.org/CONTENT/616/.

12. Joseph P. Newhouse and the Insurance Experiment Group, *Free for All? Lessons from the RAND Health Insurance Experiment* (Cambridge, Mass.: Harvard University Press, 1996), pp. 338–39.

13. Centers for Medicare & Medicaid Services, "Table 1.10—Spending for Prescription Drugs by Source of Funds, 1965–2000," *An Overview of the U.S. Healthcare System: Two Decades of Change, 1980–2000*, p. 11, http://www3.cms.hhs.gov/charts/healthcaresystem/chapter1.pdf.

14. Jalpa A. Doshi, Nicole Brandt, and Bruce Stuart, "The Impact of Drug Coverage on COX-2 Inhibitor Use in Medicare," *Health Affairs Web Exclusive*, February 18, 2004, W4–95, http://content.healthaffairs.org/cgi/reprint/hlthaff.w4.94v1.pdf.

15. This class of drugs has since come under intense scrutiny. Studies have revealed that some COX-2 inhibitors may increase the risk of stroke or serious heart attack, or may lead to potentially fatal skin reactions. At least one such drug (Vioxx) has been withdrawn from the market by its manufacturer (Merck). The FDA has requested that Pfizer pull its COX-2 inhibitor Bextra from the market as well.

16. Doshi et al., see note 14, W4-94–W4-105.

17. Carolanne Dai, Randall S. Stafford, and G. Caleb Alexander, "National Trends in Cyclooxygenase-2 Inhibitor Use since Market Release: Nonselective Diffusion of a Selectively Cost-Effective Innovation," *Archives of Internal Medicine* 165 (January 24, 2005): 175, http://home.uchicago.edu/~galexand/cox2%20paper.pdf.

18. Newhouse and the Insurance Experiment Group, see note 12.

19. Milton Friedman, "How to Cure Health Care," *The Public Interest* 142 (Winter 2001): 8–9, http://www.thepublicinterest.com/archives/2001winter/article1.html.

20. Lynne "Sam" Bishop and Bradford J. Holmes, "Who Cares about Hospital Quality Data? Plans Must Popularize Active Provider Selection," Forrester Research, October 19, 2004, http://www.forrester.com/Research/Document/Excerpt/0,7211,35295,00.html.

21. Alan C. Monheit, "Persistence in Health Expenditures in the Short Run: Prevalence and Consequences," *Medical Care* 41, no. 7, Supplement (III-56). This estimate ($1,786) is for 1997 and does not reflect subsequent growth in medical spending.

22. Lynne "Sam" Bishop and Bradford J. Holmes, "Marketing to Heart Disease Patients: Disease Differences Marketers Must Know," Forrester Research, August 31, 2004, http://www.forrester.com/Research/Document/Excerpt/0,7211,35296,00.html.

23. G. Caleb Alexander, Lawrence P. Casalino, and David O. Meltzer, "Patient-Physician Communication about Out-of-Pocket Costs," *Journal of the American Medical Association* 290, no. 7 (August 20, 2003): 953–58, http://home.uchicago.edu/%7Egalexand/costs.pdf.

24. U.S. Federal Trade Commission/Department of Justice, *Improving Health Care: A Dose of Competition*, July 23, 2004, Executive Summary, p. 6, http://www.ftc.gov/reports/healthcare/040723healthcarerpt.pdf.

25. U.S. Federal Trade Commission, "Joint FTC/Department of Justice Hearing on Health Care and Competition Law and Policy," transcript, May 27, 2003, pp. 89–90, http://www.ftc.gov/ogc/healthcarehearings/030527ftctrans.pdf.

26. Uwe E. Reinhardt, "Can Efficiency in Health Care Be Left to the Market?" *Journal of Health Policy, Politics, and Law* 26, no. 5 (October 2001): 967, 986.

27. U.S. Federal Trade Commission, "Health Care and Competition Law," transcript, March 26, 2003, p. 198, http://www.ftc.gov/ogc/healthcarehearings/030326ftctrans.pdf.

28. Regina Herzlinger, "Prix-Fixe Rip-Off," *Wall Street Journal*, June 13, 2003.

29. U.S. Federal Trade Commission/Department of Justice, see note 24, Executive Summary, p. 22.

30. U.S. Federal Trade Commission/Department of Justice, see note 24, Executive Summary, p. 5.

31. Steven M. Asch et al., "Who Is at Greatest Risk for Receiving Poor-Quality Health Care?" *New England Journal of Medicine* 354 (March 16, 2006): 1147–56.

32. Ginsburg and Nichols, see note 11.

33. Michael E. Porter and Elizabeth Teisberg, "Redefining Competition in Health Care," *Harvard Business Review*, online edition, June 1, 2004.

34. Carmen DeNavas-Walt, Bernadette D. Proctor, and Robert J. Mills, "Income, Poverty and Health Insurance Coverage in the United States: 2003," *Current Population Reports: Consumer Income*, P60-226, U.S. Bureau of the Census, August 2004, p. 14, http://www.census.gov/prod/2004pubs/p60-226.pdf.

35. Gary Claxton et al., *Employer Health Benefits: 2004 Annual Survey*, Kaiser Family Foundation/Health Research & Educational Trust, September 2004, p. 59, http://www.kff.org/insurance/7148/loader.cfm?url=/commonspot/security/getfile.cfm &PageID=46288.

36. Regina Herzlinger, "Let's Put Consumers in Charge of Health Care," *Harvard Business Review* 80, no. 7 (July 2002), http://hbswk.hbs.edu/item.jhtml?id=3045& t=strategy&noseek=one; excerpted in Herzlinger, "Are Consumers the Cure for Broken Health Insurance?" *HBS Working Knowledge*, August 5, 2002.

37. Julie A. Schoenman and Jacob J. Feldman, *2002 Survey of Physicians about the Medicare Program*, Project HOPE Center for Health Affairs, no. 03-1, March 2003, p. 43, http://www.medpac.gov/publications/contractor_reports/Mar03_02PhysSurv Rpt2.pdf.

38. "Trends and Indicators in the Changing Health Care Marketplace," Henry J. Kaiser Family Foundation, no. 7031, April 2004, section 6, p. 1 (http://www.kff.org/insurance/7031/ti2004-6-1.cfm), section 5, p. 9 (http://www.kff.org/insurance/7031/ti2004-5-9.cfm).

39. Quoted in William Goodman, "Canadian Health Insurance: Political Promises, Public Perceptions, Practical Problems," Georgia Public Policy Foundation, February 1992.

40. Jay Neugeboren, "Perfect Health, but for the Quintuple Bypass," *New York Times*, April 2, 2004, p. A19.

41. See, for example, Rhonda L. Rundle, "Pay-as-You-Go M.D.: The Doctor Is In, But Insurance Is Out; Maverick Physicians Skip Red Tape and Cut Charges," *Wall Street Journal*, November 6, 2003, p. A1; Robert Lowes, "No Coding, No Insurers—No Kidding," *Medical Economics*, April 23, 2004; http://www.cashcare.us/; http://www.hmno.com/; http://www.emergiclinic.com/; and http://simplecare.com/.

42. U.S. Federal Trade Commission/Department of Justice, see note 24, Executive Summary, pp. 21–22.

43. Andrew J. Rettenmaier and Thomas R. Saving, *The Economics of Medicare Reform* (Kalamazoo: W.E. Upjohn Institute for Employment Research, 2000), p. 141.

44. Porter and Teisberg, see note 33.

45. U.S. Federal Trade Commission/Department of Justice, see note 24, Executive Summary, p. 20.

Chapter 5

1. Robert J. Mills, "Health Insurance Coverage: 2003; Highlights," U.S. Bureau of the Census, last revised August 26, 2004, http://www.census.gov/hhes/hlthins/hlthin03/hlth03asc.html.

2. Gary Claxton et al., *Employer Health Benefits: 2004 Annual Survey*, Kaiser Family Foundation/Health Research & Educational Trust, September 2004, pp. 94–95, http://www.kff.org/insurance/7148/loader.cfm?url=/commonspot/security/getfile.cfm &PageID=46288.

3. Gary Claxton et al., *Employer Health Benefits: 2003 Annual Survey*, Kaiser Family Foundation/Health Research & Educational Trust, September 2003, p. 97, http://

www.kff.org/insurance/loader.cfm?url = /commonspot/security/getfile.cfm&Page ID = 20672.

4. Gary Claxton et al., *Employer Health Benefits: 2006 Annual Survey*, Kaiser Family Foundation/Health Research & Educational Trust, September 2006, p. 19, http://www.kff.org/insurance/7527/upload/7527.pdf.

5. Katherine Baicker and Amitabh Chandra, "The Labor Market Effects of Rising Health Insurance Premiums," NBER Working Paper no. 11160, February 2005, p. i, http://www.nber.org/papers/w11160.

6. Dana Goldman, Neeraj Sood, and Arleen Leibowitz, "Wage and Benefit Changes in Response to Rising Health Insurance Costs," NBER Working Paper no. 11063, January 2005, p. 1, http://www.nber.org/papers/w11063.

7. Authors' calculations from Gary Claxton et al., *Employer Health Benefits: 2006 Annual Survey*, Kaiser Family Foundation/Health Research & Educational Trust, September 2006, p. 19, http://www.kff.org/insurance/7527/upload/7527.pdf.

8. U.S. Bureau of the Census, "Historical Health Insurance Tables: Table HI-1. Health Insurance Coverage Status and Type of Coverage by Sex, Race and Hispanic Origin: 1987 to 2005," http://www.census.gov/hhes/www/hlthins/historic/hihistt1.html. This figure masks the growth in government coverage and the erosion of private health insurance.

9. U.S. Bureau of the Census, "Historical Health Insurance Tables: Table HI-6. Health Insurance Coverage Status and Type of Coverage by State—People under 65: 1987 to 2005," http://www.census.gov/hhes/www/hlthins/historic/hihistt6.html.

10. Claxton et al., see note 2, p. 69.

11. Julie A. Sakowski, Kathryn A. Phillips, Su-Ying Liang, and Jennifer S. Haas, "Willingness to Recommend a Health Plan: Who Is Dissatisfied and What Don't They Like?" *American Journal of Managed Care* 10, no. 6 (June 2004): 393–400.

12. Claxton et al., see note 2, p. 59.

13. Mark Pauly and Bradley Herring, *Pooling Health Insurance Risks* (Washington: American Enterprise Institute, 1999), p. 38.

14. Eduardo Porter, "Cost of Benefits Cited as Factor in Slump in Jobs," *New York Times*, August 19, 2004.

15. "Employment Cost Index: Constant Dollar Historical Listing," Bureau of Labor Statistics, Office of Compensation Levels and Trends, April 29, 2005, tables 2a, 5a, 8a, ftp://ftp.bls.gov/pub/suppl/eci.ecconst.txt. Figures are constant-dollar, nonseasonally adjusted data for civilian workers.

16. Sarah Reber and Laura Tyson, "Rising Health Care Costs Slow Job Growth and Reduce Wages and Job Quality," unpublished manuscript, August 19, 2004; cited in press release, "Kerry Outlines Health Care Plan to Bring Down Costs for Families, Strengthen the Economy and Create Jobs; New Report Out Today Shows Skyrocketing Health Costs Have Led to Job Loss and Falling Wages," Kerry-Edwards 2004, Inc., August 19, 2004.

17. Scott J. Adams, "Employer-Provided Health Insurance and Job Change," *Contemporary Economic Policy* 22, no. 3 (July 2004): 357–69.

18. Authors' estimate, updating 2002 estimate by Duke University professor Christopher Conover, based on Feldstein's original estimate. Christopher Conover, "Health Care Regulation: A $169 Billion Hidden Tax," Cato Institute Policy Analysis no. 527, October 4, 2004, p. 28, http://www.cato.org/pubs/pas/pa527.pdf.

19. 2002 estimate: $967 per household. Household data from U.S. Bureau of the Census, "Table HH-1. Households, by Type: 1940 to Present," June 12, 2003, p. 1, http://www.census.gov/population/socdemo/hh-fam/tabHH-1.pdf.

20. Clark Havighurst, *Health Care Choices: Private Contracts as Instruments of Health Reform* (Washington: AEI Press, 1995), p. 102.

21. Rep. Bill Thomas, Chairman, House Ways & Means Committee, "A Vision for Health Care," National Center for Policy Analysis briefing, National Press Club, Washington, D.C., February 12, 2004, http://www.ncpa.org/prs/tst/20040331bttst.htm.

22. Figures are for 2005. Maximum contribution limits and maximum out-of-pocket limits (i.e., maximum deductibles) are indexed annually. Minimum deductibles are not indexed. "Treasury and IRS Issue Indexed Amounts for Health Savings Accounts," JS-2112, U.S. Treasury, November 19, 2004, http://www.ustreas.gov/press/releases/js2112.htm.

23. HSA Insider, http://hsainsider.com/hsa_insurers.asp, accessed November 20, 2004.

24. Rhonda L. Rundle, "Kaiser to Offer Savings Accounts for Lower-Cost Health Coverage," *Wall Street Journal*, November 15, 2004, p. B6.

25. Robert Kazel, "Blues pledge nationwide expansion of HSAs," *American Medical News*, December 13, 2004.

26. "Everybody Launches an HSA for Next Year," *Health Market Survey*, no. 10, December 2004.

27. Hannah Yoo, "January 2007 Census Shows 4.5 Million People Covered by HSA/High-Deductible Health Plans," America's Health Insurance Plans, April 2007, http://www.ahipresearch.org/PDFs/FINAL%20AHIP_HSAReport.pdf; and "Over 10 Million Americans Now in CDH Accounts As More Companies Go over the 100,000 Mark," *Consumer Driven Market Report*, Interpro Publications, March 6, 2007.

28. "NABE Panel to Next President: Concentrate on Terror, not Stimulus," *National Association for Business Economics Economic Policy Survey*, August 17, 2004, p. 2, http://www.nabe.com/publib/pol/04/pol0408.pdf. The NABE Economic Policy Survey presents the consensus of a panel of 172 members of the National Association for Business Economics. Conducted semiannually, this survey was taken July 23–August 5, 2004.

29. Letter to Michael F. Cannon from John F. Sheils, The Lewin Group, January 7, 2005; authors' files.

30. Alan C. Monheit, "Persistence in Health Expenditures in the Short Run: Prevalence and Consequences," *Medical Care* 41, no. 7, Supplement (2003): III-56. Data are for 1997.

31. See U.S. House of Representatives Committee on Ways and Means, "Medical Security through Savings," press release, June 26, 2003, http://waysandmeans.house.gov/News.asp?FormMode=print&ID=92; and H. Rept. 108-177, to accompany H.R. 2351, "Health Savings Account Availability Act," Part 2, June 25, 2003, http://waysandmeans.house.gov/media/pdf/hr2351/hr2351commrpt.pdf.

Chapter 6

1. U.S. Federal Trade Commission/Department of Justice, *Improving Health Care: A Dose of Competition*, July 23, 2004, ch. 3, p. 29, http://www.ftc.gov/reports/healthcare/040723healthcarerpt.pdf.

2. Paul B. Ginsburg and Len M. Nichols, "The Health Care Cost-Coverage Conundrum: The Care We Want vs. the Care We Can Afford," Center for Studying Health System Change Commentary, Fall 2003, http://www.hschange.org/CONTENT/616/.

3. U.S. Federal Trade Commission/Department of Justice, see note 1, Executive Summary, p. 16.

4. "Price regulation, even if indirect, can distort provider responses to consumer demand and restrict consumer access to health care services." U.S. Federal Trade Commission/Department of Justice, see note 1, Executive Summary, p. 9.

5. U.S. Federal Trade Commission, "Joint FTC/Department of Justice Hearing on Health Care and Competition Law and Policy," transcript, May 29, 2003, p. 148, http://www.ftc.gov/ogc/healthcarehearings/030529ftctrans.pdf.

6. U.S. Federal Trade Commission/Department of Justice, see note 1, ch. 3, p. 25.

7. Ibid., Executive Summary, p. 16.

8. Uwe E. Reinhardt, "The Medicare World from Both Sides: A Conversation with Tom Scully," *Health Affairs* 22, no. 6 (November/December 2003): 168, http://content.healthaffairs.org/cgi/reprint/22/6/167.pdf.

9. "Health care markets have numerous cross-subsidies and indirect subsidies. Competitive markets compete away the higher prices and supra-competitive profits necessary to sustain such subsidies." U.S. Federal Trade Commission/Department of Justice, see note 1, Executive Summary, p. 23.

10. Jeff Tieman, "Specialty Competition Isn't All Bad: MedPAC," *ModernHealth Care.com*, September 10, 2004, http://www.modernhealthcare.com/news.cms?newsId=2885&potId=FS.

11. U.S. Federal Trade Commission/Department of Justice, see note 1, Executive Summary, p. 23.

12. Ibid., Executive Summary, pp. 19, 23.

13. *2004 Annual Report of the Board of Trustees of the Federal Hospital Insurance and Federal Supplementary Medical Insurance Trust Funds*, "Table I.C1—Medicare Data for Calendar Year 2003," (Washington: Government Printing Office, March 23, 2004), p. 3, http://www.cms.hhs.gov/publications/trusteesreport/2004/tr.pdf.

14. Sue A. Blevins, *Medicare's Midlife Crisis* (Washington: Cato Institute, 2001), p. 3.

15. John S. Hoff, *Medicare Private Contracting: Paternalism or Autonomy* (Washington: American Enterprise Institute, 1998), p. 65.

16. Blevins, see note 14, p. 42.

17. For an example of benefits changing with personnel changes, see Sarah Lueck, "Dr. McClellan's Medicare Rx," *Wall Street Journal*, September 28, 2004, http://online.wsj.com/article_print/0,,SB109632936475929585,00.html.

18. Elliott S. Fisher et al., "The Implications of Regional Variations in Medicare Spending, Part 2: Health Outcomes and Satisfaction with Care," *Annals of Internal Medicine* 138, no. 4 (February 18, 2003): 288–98, http://www.annals.org/cgi/reprint/138/4/288.pdf.

19. Jonathan Skinner, Elliott S. Fisher, and John E. Wennberg. *The Efficiency of Medicare*, NBER Working Paper no. 8395, 2001, http://dsl.nber.org/papers/w8395.pdf.

20. Estimated Medicare spending in 2007: $428 billion. U.S. Congressional Budget Office, *The Budget and Economic Outlook: Fiscal Years 2008 to 2017*, January 2007, p. 50, http://www.cbo.gov/ftpdocs/77xx/doc7731/01-24-BudgetOutlook.pdf.

21. Out of 40 indicators studied. Steven M. Asch et al., "Measuring Underuse of Necessary Care among Elderly Medicare Beneficiaries Using Inpatient and Outpatient Claims," *Journal of the American Medical Association* 284, no. 18 (November 8, 2000): 2325–33.

22. Bruce Pyenson, Steve Cigich, Kate Fitch, Troy Filipek, and Kosuke Iwasaki, "Controlling Hypertension among Medicare Beneficiaries: Saving Lives without Additional Cost," Milliman Consultants and Actuaries, September 2004, http://www.phrma.org/publications/policy//2004-08-23.1047.pdf. This study was commissioned by the Pharmaceutical Research and Manufacturers of America. Of course, the drug industry has a financial interest in encouraging greater use of antihypertensive drugs. Nonetheless, Milliman's reputation and the uneven quality delivered to Medicare patients lend plausibility to such claims.

23. Katherine Baicker and Amitabh Chandra, "Medicare Spending, the Physician Workforce, and Beneficiaries' Quality of Care," *Health Affairs Web Exclusive*, April 7, 2004, pp. W4-187, 192, http://content.healthaffairs.org/cgi/content/full/hlthaff.w4.184v1/DC1.

24. Ibid., p. W4-190, http://content.healthaffairs.org/cgi/reprint/hlthaff.w4.184v1.pdf.

25. U.S. Federal Trade Commission/Department of Justice, see note 1, ch. 3, p. 30.

26. Ibid., Executive Summary, p. 16.

27. Medicare Payment Advisory Committee, *Report to Congress: Variation and Innovation in Medicare* 108 (2003), p. 108, http://www.medpac.gov/publications/congressional_reports/June03_Entire_Report.pdf.

28. Blevins, see note 14, p. 55.

29. *2004 Annual Report of the Board of Trustees of the Federal Hospital Insurance and Federal Supplementary Medical Insurance Trust Funds* (Washington: Government Printing Office, March 23, 2004), p. 34, http://www.cms.hhs.gov/publications/trusteesreport/tr2004.pdf

30. *2007 Annual Report of the Board of Trustees of the Federal Hospital Insurance and Federal Supplementary Medical Insurance Trust Funds* (Washington: Government Printing Office, April 23, 2007), p. 27, http://www.cms.hhs.gov/ReportsTrustFunds/downloads/tr2007.pdf.

31. *2005 Annual Report of the Board of Trustees of the Federal Hospital Insurance and Federal Supplementary Medical Insurance Trust Funds* (Washington: Government Printing Office, March 23, 2005), p. 57, http://www.cms.hhs.gov/publications/trusteesreport/tr2005.pdf.

32. International Monetary Fund, World Economic Outlook Database, April 2007, http://www.imf.org/external/pubs/ft/weo/2007/01/index.htm.

33. Ibid.

34. Unfunded Social Security obligation: $15.6 trillion. *The 2007 Annual Report of the Board of Trustees of the Federal Old-Age and Survivors Insurance and Disability Insurance Trust Funds* (Washington: Government Printing Office, April 23, 2007), p. 61, http://www.ssa.gov/OACT/TR/TR07/tr07.pdf.

35. *2007 Annual Report of the Board of Trustees of the Federal Hospital Insurance and Federal Supplementary Medical Insurance Trust Funds*, pp. 67, 105, 120, http://www.cms.hhs.gov/ReportsTrustFunds/downloads/tr2007.pdf.

36. Andrew J. Rettenmaier and Thomas R. Saving, "The 2004 Medicare and Social Security Trustees Report," National Center for Policy Analysis Policy Report no. 266, June 2004, p. 11.

37. Daniel Shaviro, "How Tax Cuts Feed the Beast," *New York Times*, September 21, 2004, http://www.nytimes.com/2004/09/21/opinion/21shaviro.html.

38. Robert J. Samuelson, "Who Will Say No? Retirement Benefit Costs Are Out of Control," *Washington Post*, December 15, 2004, p. A33, http://www.washingtonpost.com/wp-dyn/articles/A134-2004Dec14.html.

39. Steve Croft, "U.S. Heading for Financial Trouble? Comptroller Says Medicare Program Endangers Financial Stability," *60 Minutes* (CBS), March 4, 2007, http://www.cbsnews.com/stories/2007/03/01/60minutes/main2528226.shtml.

40. Rettenmaier and Saving, see note 36, p. 10.

41. Thomas R. Saving, "Perspectives on the 2005 Social Security and Medicare Trustees Reports," presentation at a National Center for Policy Analysis briefing *Analyzing the 2005 Social Security and Medicare Trustees Reports,* March 23, 2005, p. 9, http://www.ncpa.org/evn/washington/2005-perspectives.pdf?PHPSESSID=f250e964d185e64ba252a97bfaed5562.

42. Personal correspondence with Jagadeesh Gokhale, November 2, 2004. Copy in authors' files.

43. Martin Feldstein, "Prefunding Medicare," National Bureau of Economic Research Working Paper no. 6917, January 1999, p. 3.

44. Ibid.

45. Elliott S. Fisher, "More Medicine Is Not Better Medicine," *New York Times,* December 1, 2003, p. A25.

46. For more on this approach, see Andrew J. Rettenmaier and Thomas R. Saving, "Reforming Medicare," National Center for Policy Analysis Policy Report no. 261, May 2003, http://www.ncpa.org/pub/st/st261/st261.pdf.

47. "All amounts are in constant 2004 dollars, adjusted to present value at age 65 using 2 percent real interest rate." C. Eugene Steuerle and Adam Carasso, "The *USA Today* Lifetime Social Security and Medicare Benefits Calculator: Assumptions and Methods," Urban Institute, October 1, 2004, http://www.urban.org/url.cfm?ID=900746 and http://www.urban.org/900746_USAToday/900746_Tables.xls.

48. Andrew J. Rettenmaier and Thomas R. Saving, *The Economics of Medicare Reform* (Kalamazoo: W.E. Upjohn Institute for Employment Research, 2000), p. 140.

49. Feldstein, see note 43, abstract and p. 10.

50. Rettenmaier and Saving, see note 48.

51. Ibid., p. 137.

52. Laurence J. Kotlikoff and Scott Burns, *The Coming Generational Storm: What You Need to Know about America's Economic Future* (Cambridge: MIT Press, 2004), p. 171.

53. In addition to the 50 states and the District of Columbia, the following territories operate their own Medicaid programs: American Samoa, Guam, the Northern Mariana Islands, Puerto Rico, and the U.S. Virgin Islands.

54. "For example, the states are prohibited by federal law from charging beneficiaries more than nominal copayments for services . . ." Jeanne M. Lambrew, "Making Medicaid a Block Grant Program: An Analysis of the Implications of Past Proposals," *Milbank Quarterly* 83, no. 1 (January 26, 2005): 44, http://www.milbank.org/quarterly/8301feature.pdf.

55. Donald B. Marron, acting director, Congressional Budget Office, Testimony before the Senate Special Committee on Aging, 109th Cong., 2d sess., July 13, 2006, p. 5, http://www.cbo.gov/ftpdocs/73xx/doc7387/07-13-Medicaid.pdf.

56. "The Medicaid Program at a Glance," Kaiser Commission on Medicaid and the Uninsured, March 2007, http://www.kff.org/medicaid/upload/7235-02.pdf.

57. Donna Cohen Ross and Laura Cox, "Beneath the Surface: Barriers Threaten to Slow Progress on Expanding Health Coverage of Children and Families," Kaiser Commission on Medicaid and the Uninsured, October 2004, p. 2, http://www.kff.org/medicaid/loader.cfm?url=/commonspot/security/getfile.cfm&PageID=47039.

58. National Association of State Budget Officers, "2005 State Expenditure Report," November 2006, pp. 2–3, http://www.nasbo.org/Publications/PDFs/2005%20State%20Expenditure%20Report.pdf.

59. Ibid., pp. 2, 47.

60. Ibid., p. 46.

61. See generally Frédéric Bastiat, *Selected Essays on Political Economy* (Irvington-on-Hudson, NY: Foundation for Economic Education, 1995), pp. 1–50.

62. Lee Anne Fennell, "Interdependence and Choice in Distributive Justice: The Welfare Conundrum," *Wisconsin Law Review* 235 (1994): 311–12.

63. This estimate is less than scientific. A number of differences between these programs might forbid applying the overconsumption estimates of Medicare to Medicaid. For example, as noted earlier, Medicaid patients are much younger than Medicare patients. Having less interaction with the health care system generally, they presumably would have fewer opportunities to overutilize care. On the other hand, cost-sharing requirements in each program may leave Medicare patients more sensitive to price. To be conservative, the number presented represents one-sixth of Medicaid spending for 2005, rather than one-fifth. What is important about this figure is not its precision but its order of magnitude.

64. Stephen Zuckerman, Joshua McFeeters, Peter Cunningham, and Len Nichols, "Changes In Medicaid Physician Fees, 1998–2003: Implications for Physician Participation," *Health Affairs Web Exclusive*, June 23, 2004, p. W4-374, http://content.healthaffairs.org/cgi/reprint/hlthaff.w4.374v1.pdf.

65. Matthew K. Wynia, Deborah S. Cummins, Jonathan B. VanGeest, and Ira B. Wilson, "Physician manipulation of reimbursement rules for patients: between a rock and a hard place," *Journal of the American Medical Association* 283, no. 14 (April 12, 2000): 1864.

66. Mark Duggan and Fiona Scott Morton, "The Distortionary Effects of Government Procurement: Evidence from Medicaid Prescription Drug Purchasing," NBER Working Paper no. 10930, November 2004, http://www.nber.org/papers/w10930.

67. Aaron S. Yelowitz, "Evaluating the Effects of Medicaid on Welfare and Work: Evidence from the Past Decade," Employment Policies Institute, December 2000, p. iv, http://epionline.org/studies/yelowitz_12-2000.pdf.

68. Ibid., p. 9.

69. Ibid., p. 4. For an example of how this disincentive affects work decisions, see Philip Dawdy, "Give Them Shelter," *Seattle Weekly*, May 5, 2004, p. 22.

70. Jonathan Gruber and Aaron Yelowitz, "Public Health Insurance and Private Savings," *The Journal of Political Economy* 107, no. 6, part 1 (December 1999): 1249–74.

71. David T. Beito, *From Mutual Aid to the Welfare State: Fraternal Societies and Social Services, 1890–1967* (Chapel Hill: University of North Carolina Press, 2000), p. 2.

72. Ibid., p. 203.

73. Ibid., p. 198.

74. Recent research corroborates that free clinics have a crowd-out effect on private health insurance. Anthony T. Lo Sasso and Bruce D. Meyer, "The Health Care Safety Net and Crowd-Out of Private Health Insurance," Joint Center for Poverty Research Working Paper, May 2003, p. 18, http://www.jcpr.org/conferences/health_policy/losasso_meyer.pdf. This suggests that Medicaid is not the only part of the medical safety net that discourages self-sufficiency.

75. Gestur Davidson et al., "Public program crowd-out of private coverage: What are the issues?" Robert Wood Johnson Foundation Research Synthesis Report no. 5, June 2004, http://www.rwjf.org/publications/synthesis/reports_and_briefs/pdf/no5_researchreport.pdf. This survey reports on 22 studies examining crowd-out of

public insurance, with results ranging from no evidence of crowd-out to crowd-out levels as high as 177 percent of increased enrollment in public programs.

76. Jeffrey R. Brown and Amy Finkelstein, "The Interaction of Public and Private Insurance: Medicaid and the Long-Term Care Insurance Market," NBER Working Paper no. 10989, December 2004, pp. 2–3, http://www.nber.org/papers/w10989.

77. Amy J. Davidoff, Bowen Garrett, and Alshadye Yemane, "Medicaid-Eligible Adults Who Are Not Enrolled: Who Are They and Do They Get the Care They Need?" Urban Institute Policy Brief, series A, no. A-48, October 1, 2001, p. 2, http://www.urban.org/url.cfm?ID=310378; and Amy J. Davidoff, Bowen Garrett, and Matthew Schirmer, "Children Eligible for Medicaid but Not Enrolled: How Great a Policy Concern?" Urban Institute Policy Brief, series A, no. A-41, September 1, 2000, pp. 1–2, http://www.urban.org/url.cfm?ID=309643.

78. Katherine Baicker and Douglas Staiger, "Fiscal Shenanigans, Targeted Federal Health Care Funds, and Patient Mortality," NBER Working Paper no. 10440, April 2004, p. 1, http://dsl.nber.org/papers/w10440.pdf; Teresa A. Coughlin, Leighton Ku, and Johnny Kim, "Reforming the Medicaid Disproportionate Share Hospital Program," Health Care Financing Review 22, no. 2 (Winter 2000): 1, http://www.cms.hhs.gov/review/00winter/00Winterpg137.pdf; and General Accounting Office, "Medicaid: State Financing Schemes Again Drive Up Federal Payments," Statement of Kathryn G. Allen before the Senate Committee on Finance, GAO/T-HEHS-00-193, September 6, 2000.

79. Mark Duggan, "Hospital Ownership and Public Medical Spending," NBER Working Paper no. 7789, July 2000, http://www.nber.org/papers/w7789.

80. Coughlin et al., see note 78.

81. Baicker and Staiger, see note 78.

82. Mark Duggan, see note 79.

83. Ibid.

84. Baicker and Staiger, see note 78, p. 30.

85. Generally, those with higher incomes pay for a larger share of Medicaid spending as a result of greater consumption and higher marginal income tax rates. However, the tax burden that Medicaid places on low-income earners cannot be taken lightly. Forty-three percent of Medicaid revenues come from state governments. Sales taxes are widely considered regressive in that relative to income, they place a larger burden on lower-income earners. On average, states rely on sales taxes for one-third of their revenue. National Association of State Budget Officers, see note 58, pp. 16, 94. In addition, state income taxes also place a significant burden on low-income families. See Joseph Llobrera and Robert Zahradnik, "The Impact of State Income Taxes on Low-Income Families in 2004," Center on Budget and Policy Priorities, April 12, 2005, http://www.cbpp.org/4-12-05sfp.pdf.

86. Julie A. Sakowski, Kathryn A. Phillips, Su-Ying Liang, and Jennifer S. Haas, "Willingness to Recommend a Health Plan: Who Is Dissatisfied and What Don't They Like?" American Journal of Managed Care, 10, no. 6 (June 2004): 393–400.

87. Zuckerman et al., see note 64.

88. Ibid., p. W4-379.

89. Julie A. Schoenman and Jacob J. Feldman, 2002 Survey of Physicians about the Medicare Program, Project HOPE Center for Health Affairs, no. 03-1, March 2003, p. 43, http://www.medpac.gov/publications/contractor_reports/Mar03_02PhysSurvRpt2.pdf.

90. "Medicaid's Role for Women," Kaiser Family Foundation Issue Brief no. 7213, November 2004, http://www.kff.org/womenshealth/loader.cfm?url=/commonspot/security/getfile.cfm&PageID=48681.

91. Alina Salganicoff and J. Zoë Beckerman, "Women's Health in the United States: Health Coverage and Access to Care," Kaiser Family Foundation, May 2002, p. 40.

92. Robert Kaestner, Theodore Joyce, and Andrew Racine, "Does Publicly Provided Health Insurance Improve the Health of Low-Income Children in the United States?" NBER Working Paper no. 6887, January 1999, p. 1, http://papers.nber.org/papers/w6887.pdf.

93. Ibid., p. 2.

94. Ibid., p. 21.

95. Ibid., p. 21.

96. Ibid., p. 22.

97. Jay Bhattacharya, Dana Goldman, and Neeraj Sood, "The Link between Public and Private Insurance and HIV-Related Mortality," NBER Working Paper no. 9346, November 2002, p. i, http://dsl.nber.org/papers/w9346.pdf.

98. Ibid., p. 14.

99. Helen Levy and David Meltzer, "What Do We Really Know about Whether Health Insurance Affects Health?" in *Health Policy and the Uninsured*, ed. Catherine McLaughlin (Washington: Urban Institute Press, 2004), p. 201. Emphasis added.

100. "The Children's Defense Fund claimed that welfare reform would cast millions of children into poverty and hunger. The Urban Institute predicted that the welfare law would cause the incomes of 1 out of 10 American families to fall and throw 1.1 million children into poverty." Robert E. Rector, "Despite Recession, Black Child Poverty Plunges to All-Time Historic Low," Heritage Foundation Backgrounder no. 1595, September 27, 2002, http://www.heritage.org/Research/Welfare/loader.cfm?url=/commonspot/security/getfile.cfm&PageID=24982.

101. U.S. Census Bureau, "Historical Poverty Tables, Table 2. Poverty Status of People by Family Relationship, Race, and Hispanic Origin: 1959 to 2005," http://www.census.gov/hhes/www/poverty/histpov/hstpov2.html.

102. *The Budget and Economic Outlook: Fiscal Years 2007 to 2017* (Washington: Congressional Budget Office, January 2007), pp. 50, 102, 106; *An Analysis of the President's Budgetary Proposals for Fiscal Year 2008* (Washington: Congressional Budget Office, March 2007), p. 47; and authors' calculations.

103. Patrick Guinane, "Daniels Signs Health Care Plan," *Northwest Indiana Times*, May 11, 2007, http://www.thetimesonline.com/articles/2007/05/11/news/top_news/doc1d6821552b40bcae862572d700835657.txt. "Medicaid HSAs Unveiled in New Hampshire," and "Five States Interested in Medicaid HSAs So Far," *Consumer Driven Market Report*, no. 9, November 2004, p. 2.

104. See, for example, James Frogue, "The Future of Medicaid: Consumer-Directed Care," Heritage Foundation Backgrounder no. 1618, January 16, 2003, http://www.heritage.org/research/healthcare/bg1618.cfm.

105. See Jim Frogue, "Medicaid's Perverse Incentives," *The State Factor*, American Legislative Exchange Council, July 2004, pp. 6–7, http://www.alec.org/meSWFiles/pdf/0420.pdf.

106. Linda Giannarelli, Paul Johnson, Sandi Nelson, and Meghan Williamson, "TRIM3's 2001 Baseline Simulation of Medicaid and SCHIP Eligibility and Enrollment: Methods and Results," Urban Institute, TRIM3 Microsimulation Project Technical

Paper, April 2005, p. 16, http://aspe.hhs.gov/health/reports/05/medicaid-schip-simulation/report.pdf.

107. Frogue, see note 105.

108. George J. Borjas, "Welfare Reform, Labor Supply, and Health Insurance in the Immigrant Population," Economic Research Initiative on the Uninsured Working Paper no. 16, May 2003, pp. 31–32, http://www.umich.edu/~eriu/pdf/wp16.pdf.

Chapter 7

1. Christopher Conover, "Health Care Regulation: A $169 Billion Hidden Tax," Cato Institute Policy Analysis no. 527, October 4, 2004, http://www.cato.org/pubs/pas/pa527.pdf. Conover's is a groundbreaking and ongoing effort to quantify the aggregate costs and benefits of health care regulation. As adjustments are made to his methodology (by Conover and others) and health care regulations, this estimate may increase or decrease.

2. Environmental Protection Agency, "Guidelines for Preparing Economic Analyses," 2000, p. 113; quoted in Conover, see note 1, p. 5.

3. Conover, see note 1, p. 20.

4. "The operation itself—the helicopters, the tanks, the fuel needed to run them, the combat pay for enlisted troops, the salaries of reservists and contractors, the rebuilding of Iraq—is costing more than $300 million a day, estimates Scott Wallsten, an economist in Washington." David Leonhardt, "What $1.2 Trillion Can Buy," *New York Times*, January 17, 2007, http://www.nytimes.com/2007/01/17/business/17leonhardt.html.

5. Kenneth D. Kochanek and Betty L. Smith, "Deaths: Preliminary Data for 2002," *National Vital Statistics Reports* (Centers for Disease Control) 52, no. 13 (February 11, 2004): 15–18, http://www.cdc.gov/nchs/data/nvsr/nvsr52/nvsr52_13.pdf.

6. National health expenditures totaled $1.5 trillion in 2002. "Table 1: National Health Expenditures Aggregate and per Capita Amounts, Percent Distribution, and Average Annual Percent Growth, by Source of Funds: Selected Calendar Years 1980–2002," Centers for Medicare & Medicaid Services, September 17, 2004, http://www.cms.hhs.gov/statistics/nhe/historical/t1.asp.

7. Conover, see note 1, p. 4.

8. Ibid., pp. 6, 11–12, 15, and authors' calculations.

9. See, for example, Peter VanDoren, "Transportation Policy," *Cato Handbook for Congress, 108th Congress*, pp. 371–73; Alfred Kahn, "Airline Deregulation," *The Concise Encyclopedia of Economics*, http://www.econlib.org/library/Enc/AirlineDeregulation.html; and Thomas Gale Moore, "Trucking Deregulation," *The Concise Encyclopedia of Economics*, http://www.econlib.org/library/Enc/TruckingDeregulation.html.

10. Victoria Craig Bunce and J. P. Wieske, "Health Insurance Mandates in the States—2004," Council for Affordable Health Insurance, July 2004, pp. 2, 7, http://www.cahi.org/cahi_contents/resources/pdf/Mandatepub2004Electronic.pdf.

11. Conover, see note 1, pp. 12–14.

12. Melinda L. Shriver and Grace-Marie Arnett, "Uninsured Rates Rise Dramatically in States with Strictest Health Insurance Regulations," Heritage Foundation Backgrounder no. 1211, August 14, 1998.

13. U.S. Federal Trade Commission/Department of Justice, *Improving Health Care: A Dose of Competition*, July 23, 2004, Executive Summary, p. 24, http://www.ftc.gov/reports/healthcare/040723healthcarerpt.pdf.

14. David Gratzer, "Less Is More: In Maryland, Deregulation Is the Bold New Idea," *National Review Online*, May 27, 2004, http://www.nationalreview.com/comment/gratzer200405270842.asp.

15. Conrad F. Meier, "Kentucky Gov. Fletcher Seeks Insurance Reform: Free-market health insurance makes slow comeback," *Health Care News*, May 1, 2004, http://www.heartland.org/Article.cfm?artId = 14790.

16. Conrad F. Meier, "New Hampshire: Valiantly Seeking Market Reform," *Health Care News*, September 1, 2004, http://www.heartland.org/Article.cfm?artId = 15519.

17. The federal Employee Retirement Income Security Act of 1974 creates an exception. It allows large employers to escape state regulation. Congress and the U.S. Department of Labor regulate the health benefits of employers who choose this option.

18. Letter from Rebecca Wittman, Zogby International, to Merrill Matthews, September 3, 2004, http://www.cahi.org/cahi_contents/resources/pdf/CAHIZogby report20040930.pdf. The poll had a margin of error of + / − 3.2 percentage points.

19. "Health Care Choice Act (H.R. 4662)," introduced June 23, 2004, http://thomas.loc.gov/cgi-bin/query/z?c108:H.R.4662:.

20. Justin Kaplan, ed., *Bartlett's Familiar Quotations*, 16th Ed. (Boston: Little, Brown and Company, 1992), p. 343.

21. Donna St. George, "Time in a Bottle: A new generation of precision cancer drugs is seducing patients with the possibility of adding months, even years, to their lives. If only they could get their hands on them," *Washington Post Magazine*, January 18, 2004, p. W10.

22. Testimony of Frank Burroughs for Hearing on Access to Experimental Drugs for the Terminally Ill, U.S. House of Representatives Committee on Government Reform, June 20, 2001, http://www.abigail-alliance.org/testimony.htm.

23. James A. Bonner et al., "Cetuximab prolongs survival in patients with locoregionally advanced squamous cell carcinoma of head and neck: A phase III study of high-dose radiation therapy with or without cetuximab (Abstract No: 5507)," *Journal of Clinical Oncology, 2004 ASCO Annual Meeting Proceedings (Post-Meeting Edition)* 22, no. 14S (July 15, 2004): 5507, http://www.asco.org/ac/1,1003,_12-002643-00_18-0026-00_19-002132,00.asp.

24. St. George, see note 21.

25. See http://www.abigail-alliance.org, and *Abigail Alliance for Better Access to Developmental Drugs et al. v. Mark B. McClellan et al.,* U.S. District Court for the District of Columbia, Civil Action no. 03-1601 (RMU), August 30, 2004, http://www.wlf.org/upload/083004DDCOpinion.pdf. The district court dismissed the case. Petitioners plan to appeal.

26. Henry I. Miller, "Failed FDA Reform," *Regulation* 21, no. 3 (1998): 24, http://www.cato.org/pubs/regulation/regv21n3/v21n3-ftr2.pdf.

27. Joseph A. DiMasi, Ronald W. Hansen, and Henry G. Grabowski, "The Price of Innovation: New Estimates of Drug Development Costs," *Journal of Health Economics* 22, no. 2 (2003): 151–85. Figures are in constant 2004 dollars.

28. Steven Neil Wiggins, "Product Quality Regulation and New Drug Introductions: Some New Evidence from the 1970s," *Review of Economic Statistics* 63 (November 1981): 615–19, and "The Impact of Regulation on Pharmaceutical Research Expenditures: A Dynamic Approach," *Economic Inquiry* 21, (January 1983): 115–28. Cited in Dale H. Gieringer, "The Safety and Efficacy of New Drug Approval," *Cato Journal* 5, no. 1 (Spring/Summer 1985): 177–201, http://www.cato.org/pubs/journal/cj5n1/cj5n1-10.pdf.

29. Editorial, "Evaluating Vioxx," *Washington Post*, October 14, 2004, p. A30, http://www.washingtonpost.com/wp-dyn/articles/A31107-2004Oct13.html.

30. Noel D. Campbell, "Making Drugs Safe and Available without the FDA," National Center for Policy Analysis Policy Report no. 208, January 1997, pp. 3–4, http://www.ncpa.org/studies/s208/s208.html.

31. Michael F. Cannon, "Aspirin Fights Heart Attacks, and the FDA Fights to Hide That Information from Your Doctor," Citizens for a Sound Economy Foundation *Capitol Comment* no. 149, November 12, 1996.

32. Gieringer, see note 28. Though somewhat dated, Conover describes Gieringer's estimates as the "most thorough empirical analysis I was able to locate." Conover, see note 1, p. 15.

33. See Sam Peltzman, "An Evaluation of Consumer Protection Legislation: The 1962 Drug Amendments," *Journal of Political Economy* 81, no. 5 (1973): 1049–91; Dale H. Gieringer, "The Safety and Efficacy of New Drug Approval," *Cato Journal* 5, no. 1 (Spring/Summer 1985): 177–201; Mary K. Olson, "Are Novel Drugs More Risky for Patients Than Less Novel Drugs?" *Journal of Health Economics* 23 (2004): 1135–1158; Tomas J. Philipson et al., "Assessing the Safety and Efficacy of the FDA: The Case of the Prescription Drug User Fee Acts," NBER Working Paper no. 11724, October 2005.

34. Conover, see note 1, p. 15.

35. The activists who mobilized to speed the approval of new AIDS drugs and the Abigail Alliance are rare exceptions that offer visibility to a few victims.

36. Former FDA commissioner Alexander Schmidt, quoted in Sam Kazman, "Deadly Overcaution: FDA's Drug Approval Process," *Journal of Regulation and Social Costs* 1, no. 1 (September 1990): 41, http://www.cei.org/pdf/3887.pdf.

37. Henry I. Miller, *To America's Health: A Proposal to Reform the Food and Drug Administration* (Stanford: Hoover Institution Press, 2000), pp. 41–42.

38. Ibid., pp. 21–22.

39. See Mary K. Olson, "How Have User Fees Affected the FDA?" *Regulation* 25, no. 1 (Spring 2002): 20–25, http://www.cato.org/pubs/regulation/regv25n1/v25n1-2.pdf.

40. See Daniel B. Klein and Alexander Tabarrok, "Who Certifies Off-Label?" *Regulation* 27, no. 2 (Summer 2004): 60–63, http://www.cato.org/pubs/regulation/regv27n2/v27n2-8.pdf.

41. J. Howard Beales III, "New Uses for Old Drugs," in Robert B. Helms, ed., *Competitive Strategies in the Pharmaceutical Industry*, American Enterprise Institute, 1996, p. 303. The study looked at citations in the *U.S. Pharmacopoeia Drug Information*, "an authoritative compendium of drug information."

42. Former FDA deputy commissioner for policy William B. Schultz, "How to Improve Drug Safety," *Washington Post*, December 2, 2004, p. A35, http://www.washingtonpost.com/wp-dyn/articles/A26865-2004Dec1.html.

43. All are found or derived from "National Data," Organ Procurement and Transplantation Network, June 22, 2007 (current waiting lists accessed June 29, 2007), http://www.optn.org/data/.

44. "National Data," see note 43.

45. Ibid.

46. David J. Theroux et al., *An Open Letter from 539 Economists from All 50 States on Health Care Policy Reform*, The Independent Institute, March 1, 2000, http://www.independent.org/newsroom/article.asp?id=490.

47. David L. Kaserman and A. H. Barnett, *The U.S. Organ Procurement System: A Prescription for Reform* (Washington: American Enterprise Institute, 2002), pp. 114–15.

48. Nancy Sheper-Hughes, "Organs without Borders," *Foreign Policy*, January/February 2005, p. 27, http://www.foreignpolicy.com/Ning/archive/archive/146/PN146.pdf.

49. To be sure, the provider is more vulnerable to kidney failure as a result of having only one kidney. One way to protect against this risk would be for recipients to purchase insurance to cover any future medical care the provider may need as a result of the operation.

50. It bears noting that Americans who decry queue-jumping by elites in nations with socialized medicine often fail to recognize it at home.

51. Christopher Windham, "Blacks Urged to Help Close Gap in Availability of Donor Organs," *Wall Street Journal*, November 24, 2004, p. D4.

52. Lloyd R. Cohen, "Directions for the Disposition of My (and Your) Vital Organs," *Regulation* 28, no. 3 (Fall 2005): 32–38, http://www.cato.org/pubs/regulation/regv28n3/v28n3-1.pdf.

53. LifeSharers is an organization that seeks to increase the supply of donated organs by offering a nonmonetary incentive to donate. Anyone can join LifeSharers and membership is free. Each member agrees to be an organ donor, and directs that other LifeSharers members are first in line to obtain his or her organs. If no LifeSharers member needs them, they become available to nonmembers. In exchange, LifeSharers members in need of an organ transplant get first access to any "LifeSharers organs" that become available. In essence, the reward for agreeing to donate when you die is a better chance of getting an organ if you ever need one to live. See http://www.lifesharers.com/.

54. The payment could come from the patient needing the transplant, or anyone else on that patient's behalf. Cohen notes this sum is "a bit more than 1% of the initial cost of a renal transplant and considerably less than that for the other organ grafts." He hopes the proceeds from the "modest" price he asks for "these irreplaceable life-saving organs" would go toward "a nice but not extravagant party celebrating my life." Cohen, see note 52, p. 2.

55. Citing Freedman, "The Ethical Continuity of Transplantation," *Transplantation Proceedings* 17, no. 23, supp. IV (1985): Cohen, see note 52, p. 15.

56. "Mark Twain, Osteopath, Appears at Public Hearing Before Assembly Committee; His Personal Liberty Plea: Wants to Try Everything That Comes Along—Adam, He Says, Was Unjustly Criticized," *New York Times*, February 28, 1901, http://www.twainquotes.com/19010228.html.

57. U.S. Federal Trade Commission/Department of Justice, *Improving Health Care: A Dose of Competition*, July 23, 2004, Executive Summary, p. 14, http://www.ftc.gov/reports/healthcare/040723healthcarerpt.pdf.

58. See, for example, Pamela Venning et al., "Randomised controlled trial comparing cost-effectiveness of general practitioners and nurse practitioners in primary care," *British Medical Journal* 320 (April 15, 2000): 1048–53, and Walter O. Spitzer et al., "The Burlington Randomized Trial of the Nurse Practitioner," *The New England Journal of Medicine* 290, no. 5 (January 31, 1974): 251–56.

59. U.S. Federal Trade Commission/Department of Justice, see note 57, ch. 2, p. 28.

60. Morris M. Kleiner, "Occupational Licensing," *Journal of Economic Perspectives* 14, no. 4 (Fall 2000): 190.

61. "Empirical studies have found that licensing regulation increases costs for consumers." U.S. Federal Trade Commission/Department of Justice, see note 57, ch. 2, p. 27.

62. Paul Starr, *The Social Transformation of American Medicine* (USA: Basic Books, 1982), p. 126.

63. Conover, see note 1, pp. 11–12.

64. Chris W. Paul, "Physician Licensure Legislation and the Quality of Medical Care," *Atlantic Economic Journal*, 1984, p. 27, as cited in Carolyn Cox and Susan Foster, *The Costs and Benefits of Occupational Regulation* (Washington: Federal Trade Commission, October 1990), p. 19.

65. Ha T. Tu and J. Lee Hargraves, "High Cost of Medical Care Prompts Consumers to Seek Alternatives," Center for Studying Health System Change Data Bulletin no. 28, December 2004, http://hschange.org/CONTENT/722/.

66. U.S. Congress, Office of Technology Assessment, *Nurse Practitioners, Physician Assistants, and Certified Nurse-Midwives: A Policy Analysis* (Health Technology Case Study 37), OTA-HCS-37 (Washington: U.S. Government Printing Office, December 1986), p. 29, http://www.wws.princeton.edu/cgi-bin/byteserv.prl/~ota/disk2/1986/8615/8615.PDF.

67. Institute of Medicine, *Allied Health Services: Avoiding Crises* (Washington: National Academy Press, 1989), p. 253.

68. Stanley J. Gross, "Professional Licensure and Quality: The Evidence," Cato Institute Policy Analysis no. 79, December 9, 1986, http://www.cato.org/pub_display.php?pub_id=945&full=1.

69. Ibid.

70. Tom Rademacher, "Don't Try This at Home!" *Ann Arbor News*, February 9, 1997, p. A-11; cited in Kleiner, see note 60.

71. Milton Friedman, *Capitalism and Freedom* (Chicago: University of Chicago, 2002), p. 158.

72. U.S. Federal Trade Commission/Department of Justice, see note 57, Executive Summary, p. 22.

73. Charles A. Baron, "Licensure of Health Care Professionals: The Consumer's Case for Abolition," *American Journal of Law and Medicine* 9 (1983): 351, citing Locke, Mode & Binswager, *The Case against Medical Licensing*, 8 Medicolegal News, October 1980, pp. 13–14.

74. U.S. Federal Trade Commission/Department of Justice, see note 57, Executive Summary, p. 22.

75. Ibid.

76. David Mechanic, "Physician Discontent: Challenges and Opportunities," *Journal of the American Medical Association* 290, no. 7 (August 20, 2003): 941–46.

77. U.S. Federal Trade Commission/Department of Justice, see note 57, Executive Summary, p. 22.

78. U.S. General Accounting Office, *Specialty Hospitals: Geographic Locations, Services Provided and Financial Performance*, GAO-04-167, 2003, p. 15, http://www.gao.gov/new.items/d04167.pdf.

79. See, for example, Michael Morrissey, "State Health Care Reform: Protecting the Provider," in Roger D. Feldman, ed., *American Health Care: Government, Market*

Processes, and the Public Interest (Oakland, Calif: The Independent Institute, 2000), pp. 245–48; and U.S. Federal Trade Commission/Department of Justice, see note 57, ch. 8, pp. 5–6.

80. Scott Hankins, "Certificate of Need Regulation and Health Outcomes," unpublished manuscript, January 30, 2004; Hankins is a doctoral candidate in economics at the University of Florida, http://plaza.ufl.edu/shankins/cv.htm.

81. U.S. Federal Trade Commission/Department of Justice, see note 57, Executive Summary, p. 22.

82. U.S. Office of Management and Budget, *Budget of the United States Government, Fiscal Year 2006* (Washington: Government Printing Office, 2005), p. 7.

Chapter 8

1. Christopher Conover, "Health Care Regulation: A $169 Billion Hidden Tax," Cato Institute Policy Analysis no. 527, October 4, 2004, p. 18, http://www.cato.org/pubs/pas/pa527.pdf.

2. See Michael I. Krauss and Robert A. Levy, "Can Tort Reform and Federalism Coexist?" Cato Institute Policy Analysis no. 514, April 14, 2004, http://www.cato.org/pubs/pas/pa514.pdf (rejecting the interstate commerce clause justification for federal tort reforms: "Shocking malpractice damage awards, if indeed they are systemically too high, are not commerce and seldom interstate").

3. Michael S. Greve, "Liability Reform: Carpe Diem," American Enterprise Institute Federalist Outlook no. 22, December 2004, p. 4, http://www.aei.org/docLib/20041124_no.22%2317663graphics.pdf.

4. Jonathan Klick and Thomas Stratmann, "Does Medical Malpractice Reform Help States Retain Physicians and Does It Matter?" American Enterprise Institute, September 2003, http://www.aei.org/docLib/20030910_Reform.pdf.

5. John C. Goodman and Gerald Musgrave, *Patient Power* (Washington: Cato Institute, 1992), p. 64.

6. Ibid., note 38.

7. Michael I. Krauss, "Restoring the Boundary: Tort Law and the Right to Contract," Cato Institute Policy Analysis no. 347, June 3, 1999, pp. 1, 11, http://www.cato.org/pubs/pas/pa347.pdf.

8. John Lancaster, "Surgeries, Side Trips for 'Medical Tourists'; Affordable Care at India's Private Hospitals Draws Growing Number of Foreigners," *Washington Post*, October 21, 2004, p. A1, http://www.washingtonpost.com/wp-dyn/articles/A49743-2004Oct20.html.

9. Vicki Cheng, "Americans increasingly find health care abroad," *News & Observer* (Raleigh), September 23, 2004, http://www.newsobserver.com/news/nc/v-printer/story/1664206p-7897201c.html.

Conclusion

1. See Michael F. Cannon, "Health Savings Accounts Are Crucial to Medicare Reform," National Center for Policy Analysis Brief Analysis no. 447, July 11, 2003, http://www.ncpa.org/pub/ba/ba447/ba447.pdf.

2. Michael E. Porter and Elizabeth Teisberg, "Redefining Competition in Health Care," *Harvard Business Review*, online edition, June 1, 2004.

Index

Page references followed by f denote figures.

Abigail Alliance for Better Access to Developmental Drugs, 121, 122
access to medical care, 2
  liberalizing medical licensing and, 140–41
  medical technology, comparisons, 17, 18f
acquired immunodeficiency syndrome (AIDS), mortality-to-incidence ratios, international comparison, 17, 19f
advertising, medical, 65, 123
affordability, health care, 1, 2, 14
African Americans
  mutual-aid societies and, 102–3
  waiting for transplantable organs, 132–33, 133f
aging and elderly persons
  excessive coverage prompting generational conflicts, 57
  health spending and, 20, 27
  Medicaid for, 96
AIDS care
  cost-effectiveness of anti-AIDS drugs, 22
  mortality-to-incidence ratios, international comparison, 17, 19f
  See also HIV patients
Aid to Families with Dependent Children, 101, 109
allied health professionals, 135, 141
alternative medicine, 136–37
ambulatory surgery centers (ASCs), 82
American Hospital Formulary Service Drug Information, 126, 127
American Telemedicine Association, 140
Apollo Hospitals, 8, 9
Arnett, Grace-Marie (Turner), 118
aspirin, "off-label" use, 123, 126
automobile insurance analogy, 44

Baiker, Katherine, 69, 87
Barnett, A. H., 131
barriers to entry, economic competition and, 4, 10–11, 134, 135, 138
baseball metaphor, for competition, 2–3
Beeney, Robert, 8
Beito, David, 102–3
benefit-cost ratio of health care spending, 21–22, 21f
Bernard, Louis, 103
Beth Israel Deaconess Medical Center, 55–56
birth weight, 24
Blevins, Sue, 85
BlueCross/BlueShield, 73, 85
Borjas, George, 111–13
breast cancer, mortality-to-incidence ratios, international comparison, 17, 19f
Britain
  National Health Service in, 8, 36, 37, 85
  shortages and wait for treatment, 36, 37
Brown, Jeffrey, 104
bureaucracy, health care, 10, 48
  managed care, 69–70
  Massachusetts Health Care Connector, 38–40, 43, 45, 46–47
  medical ethic and, 63
  Medicare, 85
  U.S. health care system, 29–30
Burroughs, Abigail, 121–22, 126
Burroughs, Frank, 121, 122
Bush, George W., 12, 72, 78, 143

California, employer mandates in, 42–43
Canada
  cost of single-payer health care system, 36–37, 38
  expenditures on medical care in United States by, 18
  health spending in, 38
  income taxes, 38

179

185

About the Authors

Michael F. Cannon is the Cato Institute's director of health policy studies. Previously, he served as a domestic policy analyst at the U.S. Senate Republican Policy Committee under Senator Larry E. Craig (R-ID), where he advised the Senate leadership on health, education, labor, welfare, and Second Amendment policy. In addition, Cannon has worked as a health care policy analyst for Citizens for a Sound Economy Foundation in Washington, D.C. Cannon has appeared on CNN, CNBC, C-SPAN, FOX News Channel, NPR, *The Michael Reagan Show*, and *The Alan Keyes Show*. His articles have been featured in *USA Today*, the *New York Post*, the *Chicago Tribune*, the *Chicago Sun-Times*, and the *San Francisco Chronicle*.

As director of Cato's health and welfare studies, Michael Tanner heads research on new, market-based approaches to health, welfare, and Social Security. His approach is based on individual responsibility rather than government control. A prolific author and frequent lecturer, Tanner served as director of research at the Georgia Public Policy Foundation before joining Cato in 1993. Under Tanner's direction, Cato launched the Project on Social Security Choice, widely considered the leading impetus for transforming the soon-to-be-bankrupt system into a private savings program. Most recently, Tanner has coauthored two books: *A New Deal for Social Security* and *Common Cents, Common Dreams: A Layman's Guide to Social Security Reform*. Tanner's writing has been published in the *Washington Post*, the *Los Angeles Times*, the *Wall Street Journal*, and *USA Today*. He has appeared on *The NewsHour with Jim Lehrer*, ABC, CBS, NBC, NPR, FOX News Channel, MSNBC, CNBC, C-SPAN, and Voice of America.

Cato Institute

Founded in 1977, the Cato Institute is a public policy research foundation dedicated to broadening the parameters of policy debate to allow consideration of more options that are consistent with the traditional American principles of limited government, individual liberty, and peace. To that end, the Institute strives to achieve greater involvement of the intelligent, concerned lay public in questions of policy and the proper role of government.

The Institute is named for *Cato's Letters*, libertarian pamphlets that were widely read in the American Colonies in the early 18th century and played a major role in laying the philosophical foundation for the American Revolution.

Despite the achievement of the nation's Founders, today virtually no aspect of life is free from government encroachment. A pervasive intolerance for individual rights is shown by government's arbitrary intrusions into private economic transactions and its disregard for civil liberties.

To counter that trend, the Cato Institute undertakes an extensive publications program that addresses the complete spectrum of policy issues. Books, monographs, and shorter studies are commissioned to examine the federal budget, Social Security, regulation, military spending, international trade, and myriad other issues. Major policy conferences are held throughout the year, from which papers are published thrice yearly in the *Cato Journal*. The Institute also publishes the quarterly magazine *Regulation*.

In order to maintain its independence, the Cato Institute accepts no government funding. Contributions are received from foundations, corporations, and individuals, and other revenue is generated from the sale of publications. The Institute is a nonprofit, tax-exempt, educational foundation under Section 501(c)3 of the Internal Revenue Code.

CATO INSTITUTE
1000 Massachusetts Ave., N.W.
Washington, D.C. 20001
www.cato.org